CHAIR YOGA & WALL PILATES

FOR SENIORS

(2 Books in 1)

Improve Balance, Mobility, Posture
And Heart Health

Luna Light

This book includes 2 titles:

WALL PILATES FOR SENIORS

For Weight Loss, Balance, Mobility and
Better Posture In Under 10 Min A Day

CHAIR YOGA FOR SENIORS

28-Day Challenge to Lose Weight, Improve Posture, Balance,
Mobility, & Strength in 10 Minutes a Day

DISCLAIMER

This book is intended to provide readers with general information about yoga exercises and routines. The content provided is not a substitute for professional medical advice, diagnosis, or treatment. Engaging in any exercise program carries the risk of injury. While the author and publisher have made every effort to ensure the safety of the exercises and routines described in this book, they cannot guarantee that they are appropriate for every individual. Always seek the advice of a qualified healthcare provider with any questions you may have regarding a medical condition or physical exercise regimen if you are unsure. If you experience pain, dizziness, discomfort, or any other symptoms while performing any of the exercises described in this book, stop immediately and consider seeking medical attention. By voluntarily participating in any of the exercises shown in this publication, you accept the risk of any potential injury.

Letter to You, The Reader

Congratulations. Your purchase of this book bundle includes two amazing books that help you increase your flexibility, strength and mind and body awareness all centered around Chair Yoga and Wall Pilates movements.

The first book, **Chair Yoga for Seniors** introduces new movements in the chair using the stability of a chair. This will give you variety and more movements that help improve strength if you're mobility limited. This one is easier than the first, and if you're just starting out will be great to use this and go at a slower pace.

The second book is my best seller **Wall Pilates For Seniors**. Even if you're not a senior woman, you can benefit greatly from this comprehensive book on gentle Wall Pilates movements.

As you work with the first movements you will begin to feel more lively and flexible. Listen to your body as you go and adapt. Don't be afraid to slow down and if you do speed up, do it slowly, day by day.

Some of the paragraphs may sound repetitive at first, but they are there so remind you of the fundamentals of Pilates and Yoga movements, and how to do them slowly, safely and calmly.

If you have any questions email me at luna@wallpilates.org.

Thank you for letting me be your guide in your journey to a healthy, happy and fit life.

Love,

Luna Light

Contents

LUNA LIGHT – 1

Letter to You, The Reader   3

CHAIR YOGA FOR SENIORS – 7

The Problem of Aging   8
The Solution   9
"Why Should I Listen to You, Luna?"   10
How Chair Yoga Can Help You   11
What You Need to Start   12
How To Breathe (Important!)   13
The Workout Plan   16

Balance Exercises   17
Balance Check   18
Alexander Technique (Using a Chair)   20
Alexander Technique (Standing)   22
The Monkey   26
The Sky Reach   27
Hip Circles   28

Warm-Up Exercises   29
Seated Chest Claps   30
Chair Spinal Twist   31
Chair Side Stretch   31
Chair Downward Stretch   32
Cobra Pose Chair   32
Chair Arm Circle   33

Cardio Exercises   35
Chair Leg Extension   36
Sitting Duck Pose   37
The Sparrow   37
Torso Twist   38
Chair Warrior Pose   39
Dancer Pose   40

Sitting Jacks   41

Flexibility Exercises   **43**
Chair Eagle   44
Cat Stretch & Breathwork   45
Floor Leg Raise   46
Heel Raises   46
Upward Hand Stretch   47
Chair Leg Raise   48
Chair Cat-Cow   48
Hand Stretch   49
Seated Knee Stretch   50
Chair Leg Kicks   50
Chair Half Warrior Pose   51
Standing Head Stretch   52
Seated Stretch & Bend   53
Seated Head & Arm Stretch   54
Seated Half Moon Pose   55
Chair Squat   56

Next Steps   57
Thank You   58
Additional Resources   59
Citations   59
Disclosures   59
The Legal Stuff   59

WALL PILATES FOR SENIORS — 61

Magic in Movement as We Age   63
Why Wall Pilates for Seniors?   65
What You Need to Start   69
How to Breathe When You Move   71
My Chronic Pain Story   74

Gentle Warm-Up Routine   **75**
Wall Leg Stretch   76
Wall Staff Pose   77
Shoulder Arm Stretch   78
Knee Stretch   78
Hugging Knee Pose   79
Wall Spine Stretch   80
Child's Pose   81

Checking for Trigger Points 82

Control And Balance 83
Balance Check 84
The Monkey 86
Hip Circles 87
The Wall Roll Up 88
The Spine Stretch 89
Wall Downward Dog 90
Wall Downard Facing Dog 91
Legs Up the Wall Pose 92
Straddle Pose 93
Standing Side Bend Pose 94
Garland Pose with Wall 95
Standing Backbend Pose 96
Wall Butterfly Pose 97
Wall Roll Down 98

Cardio Focus 99
Wall Leg Raise to Back Kick 100
Wall Plank 101
Leg Embrace 102
Wall Calf Raises 103
Wall Twist 104
The Backward Balance 105
Straight-Legged Sit-Ups 106
Wall Leg Swings 107
Wall Angels 108
Wall Sit-Ups 109

Next Steps 110
Additional Resources 111
Citations 111
Disclosures 111

BOOK 1

CHAIR YOGA
FOR SENIORS

*28-Day Challenge to Lose Weight,
Improve Posture, Balance, Mobility,
& Strength in 10 Minutes a Day*

The **Problem** of Aging

"Old age is a shipwreck."
— *Charles de Gaulle*

After the age of fifty, the human body experiences many changes that make it easier to gain weight, lose muscle, and have poorer posture.

It starts with a decline in testosterone and growth hormones. On average, between ages 30 and 70, testosterone declines by 1–2 percent a year. One to two percent might not sound like much, but that's a 20 percent decline by age 50 and a 40 percent decline by age 70![*] With lower testosterone, muscle mass tends to decrease, and fat mass tends to increase. Because the muscles control movements in our joints, bone health issues (osteoporosis) start occurring. Less growth hormones also mean muscle repair and recovery are slower, so workouts don't feel as fun as they used to during and afterward.

In America, our mobility and flexibility are further limited by a prolonged sedentary lifestyle and an increase in reliance on technology. Because our city infrastructure requires cars to get around, we sit around more in them instead of walking, we watch more and more TV, stare at our phones with Internet access, and over the years... our mobility starts to decline, slowly at first and faster as time accumulates.

Yet, for every case of limited mobility and dwindling health, there are 50, 60, 70, and 80-year-olds with vibrant energy who feel freedom in their movements.

My dad is 72. He plays golf on Mondays, hangs out with friends on Tuesdays, and plays the saxophone with his elder group on Wednesdays. Every morning and evening, he takes a brisk walk around his house. Mom follows him around when she feels like it. Otherwise, she's tending to her garden—digging, planting, and selling the vegetables she grows mostly for recreation.

In addition to my parents, many senior students of mine who practice yoga, Pilates, and somatic movements (low-risk, low-impact forms of exercise) with gentle movement techniques all retain their physical and mental functions despite aging bodies.

That's why if you want to feel lighter, healthier, and have more freedom with your body, you're in luck! This book will help you discover a holistic solution to rebuilding your body using chair yoga, no matter how old you are.

---

[*]   B. R. Zirkin and J. L. Tenover. "Aging and declining testosterone past, present, and hopes for the future." *Journal of Andrology.* (2012). 1111–1118. https://www.ncbi.nlm.nih.gov/pmc/articles/PMC4077344/

The Solution

"You are never too old to set another goal or to dream a new dream."
— C. S. Lewis

Chair yoga is the reason you bought this book.

But chair yoga itself is NOT the answer. Before you start looking for the refund page on Amazon, let me explain: Chair yoga is just a tool for us to get to the real solution.

What is the real solution to weight loss, limited mobility, and bad posture as we age?

In my humble opinion, it's a holistic approach of proper alignment, movement, and exercise that gives freedom to your body's movements. And in order to start this process, we're going to focus on the chair.

Why the chair? Because the chair helps us do three things really well:

First, it provides **instant feedback.** We can feel how strong we're pushing against an object, and we can add resistance training against it.

Second, the chair gives us **stability;** it's an object to stand, move, and exercise our muscles around even if we have limited mobility, whether sitting down or using it as a stabilizer while standing.

Third, the chair can help us become **aware of our spinal alignment and posture.** I'll show you how to do this using the principles of the Alexander technique in the first group of exercises.

"Why Should I Listen to You, Luna?"

"The only disability in life is a bad attitude."
— Scott Hamilton, Olympic figure skater and cancer survivor

You might be wondering who I am and why you should listen to me.

Hi, I'm Luna. I'm a Pilates and yoga teacher who recovered from a car accident using the exercises I'm about to teach you.

Five years ago, I was in an accident that left me in so much pain that I could not walk and was restricted to a small bedroom at a friend's house. Necessity forced me to discover new ways of exercising and getting my life back.

Over the next year, I started learning about ways to exercise and strengthen my body by using low-impact but highly effective training. I learned about Pilates, yoga, and somatic movements.

It took a long time, but I recovered from my chronic pain using a combination of these soothing movements. As I continued to strengthen my body, I was surprised to find that the pain was gone, and I continued to get stronger and more flexible and had better posture than I had before the accident!

Chair yoga is simple and easy, and if you're mobility-restricted offers a gentle way to strengthen your body. You can do it in the comfort of your home.

Trigger Point Check

One thing you should look into if you're not seeing improvement is to check for trigger points where you sense muscle pain or weakness. If you have active trigger points, exercising the muscle does not solve the problem. In this case, I highly recommend The Trigger Point Therapy Workbook by the late Clair Davies.

If you have trigger points, our goal is to **1)** clear any trigger points in your muscles and then **2)** use low-risk, low-impact but efficient exercise movements to regain strength. By doing it in this order, you will become tension-free and stronger.

The movements in this book only take fifteen to twenty minutes a day. And all it takes is two weeks for this to become a feel-good habit.

Love,

Luna Light

How **Chair Yoga Can** Help You

"Yoga is the journey of the self, through the self, to the self."
— The Bhagavad Gita

Chair yoga provides a solution for us to gain strength and mobility while minimizing the chance of injury by using the stabilizing force of the chair. You can do it anytime you're sitting down in the comfort of your own home. You can combine it with other forms of exercise or just do it once a day for fifteen minutes.

Why Chair Yoga?	Chair Yoga	Other Training Forms
Injury Risk	Low impact, less chance of inflammation. Stable.	Need resting days, possibility of overtraining and injuring or straining muscles.
Accessibility	People with disabilities, injuries, mobility issues, and seniors can still do all exercises safely.	For those with mobility issues, intense weight training routines can be dangerous and set you back more.
Intensity	Loving the feeling instead of "forcing it." Less burn out.	Pushing to the limit.
Fat Burn	Can still get a good workout and sweat even if mobility is limited.	Can feel exhausting or overtrained. Can't train if limited mobility.
Feeling	Feels like you're moving at your own pace, instead of under pressure or "competing."	Feels really sore after, feels fast and rushed.
Results	More tone, strength, and spinal alignment using stability of chair. Holistic and accessible.	Isolates specific muscles. Can become muscular but at the expense of holistic health.

When compared to other forms of exercise, chair yoga is safer and more convenient for seniors, rehabilitation clients, those with mobility issues, or anyone who just wants to start out slowly and comfortably.

The chair allows us to gain all these advantages without any cost.

What You Need to Start

"You don't have to be great to start, but you have to start to be great."
— Zig Ziglar

The 28-day program in this book is a guide to help you move at your own pace. It's not a race. To begin... you'll need:

1. **A sturdy chair:** It helps if your chair has four legs and is sturdy. Make sure it can sustain your weight when you lean on it, even if you push heavily. Avoid heavy, immovable chairs, chairs with no back support, and rocking chairs. We're looking for a standard, sturdy, and moveable chair.

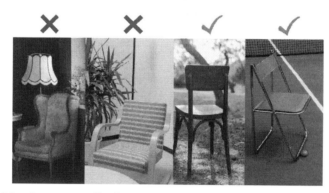

2. **A pillow, a yoga block, or a rolled-up towel** can help you soften the seat and assist as an anchor in certain exercises. This is optional.

3. **Clear space:** Ensure the area around the wall is free from obstacles, slippery rugs, glass, or loose items that could lead to trips or falls.

4. **Footwear and attire:** Wear appropriate, nonslip footwear if you prefer. Chair yoga is very effective barefoot. Comfortable, form-fitting attire can help you move freely without getting tangled or caught.

5. **Water bottle:** Drink plenty of water before, during, and after your exercise session to prevent muscle cramps and promote recovery. I always prepare a water bottle before a workout so I stay hydrated no matter what.

When exercising, if you feel like you're pushing too hard... it's okay to rest and then start again slowly. Consistency is more important than "going hard." My mentor once told me: "Being extraordinary is simply performing ordinary things consistently over a period of time."

So go at your own pace. This isn't a race... there's no competition here. Think of it as playing with your own "limitations" and expanding them beyond your current comfort zone.

How To Breathe (Important!)

"Breathing is the first act of life and the last. Our very life depends on it. Since we cannot live without breathing, it is tragically deplorable to contemplate the millions and millions who have never mastered the art of correct breathing."
— Joseph Pilates, inventor of Pilates*

The most important thing to remember is the coordination of the breath to help the movement of your body.

Practicing Breathing

Try this out. Inhale through your nose: Taking a deep breath in, aim to expand the ribcage out to the sides, allowing the lungs to fill up with air.

Now exhale through the mouth: Purse your lips as if you're blowing out through a straw and exhale fully, engaging your core muscles and feeling the abdominal wall draw inward.

How does it feel? Pretty good, right? Now, try inhaling and exhaling with your mouth fully to 100 percent limit. Do you feel your chest expanding? Lungs reaching places it hasn't gone before? Good. Now, try inhaling and exhaling with your nose. How does that feel? Chances are your nose feels smooth (more filters for pollution through the nostrils), and using your mouth feels like you have more breathing capacity.

The breath gives us so much untapped power. Practicing this increases your breathing capacity and your ability to do more movements. To increase my breathing abilities, I use visualization. When I'm practicing, I'm sitting down on the chair or lying on the floor in the corpse pose. Sometimes, I take the lightning (yoga) pose.

---

*   Joseph H. Pilates and William J. Miller. *Return to Life Through Contrology,* (Mockingbird Press, 2021).

Corpse pose:

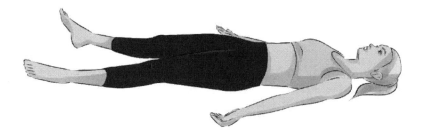

Lightning pose:

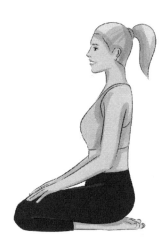

I imagine my rib cage expanding. Then I imagine my abdomen expanding, then my upper back, then my lower back. With each breath, I see if I can expand my lungs and diaphragm in all directions. This practice has improved my breathing capacity significantly after just a few months. Note that if you use your mouth to inhale and exhale, you can expand further with more air and then revert back to nose breathing on subsequent counts. When I first started, I was limited to nose breathing, which I was told is healthier (which is true), but when my teacher taught me to breathe in using my mouth, I suddenly was able to expand my chest and lungs, and I realized I was severely limited by years of nose breathing to the point where my chest wasn't even moving and my air intake was low!

Do ten minutes of this every morning and see how your breathing capacity changes in just a few short weeks.

A Sure Way to Feel Calm

The 4-7-8 technique, also known as the "relaxing breath," is a simple breathing exercise developed by Dr. Andrew Weil. It's inspired by an ancient yogic technique called *pranayama,* which involves the regulation of breath to enhance physical and mental well-being.

The 4-7-8 technique is designed to act as a natural tranquilizer for the nervous system, so it's great at the end of a workout. In fact, I use it whenever I feel rushed or stressed outside the gym.

4-7-8 Steps:

1. Inhale quietly through the nose for a count of four.

2. Hold your breath for a count of seven.

3. Exhale completely through the mouth, making a whoosh sound, for a count of eight.

This is one breath cycle. Aim to complete this cycle for four breaths while you relax.

Box Breathing

Box breathing, also known as square breathing, is a relaxation and stress reduction technique that has been utilized in various practices, including yoga, meditation, and tactical settings in the military. The best part about this is that it's easy to remember: Four seconds in, four seconds hold, four seconds out, four seconds hold.

Box breathing has been used to help soldiers and law enforcement personnel manage stress and anxiety and maintain focus in high-pressure situations. Special operations units and tactical training programs often incorporate this breathing technique as a means to enhance performance and cognitive control. The technique itself—employing a pattern of controlled breaths in a four-part sequence—has deep roots in ancient practices, especially in disciplines such as yoga and meditation. Pranayama, the yogic practice of breath control, features various breathing exercises, some of which resemble the box breathing technique. These ancient practices aim to regulate and control the breath to improve physical, mental, and emotional well-being. Here are the practice instructions:

Breathing Pattern: Follow this sequence for each breath phase:

- **Inhale (4 seconds):** Breathe in slowly and deeply through your nose for a count of four seconds. Feel your lungs expanding as you do so.

- **Hold (4 seconds):** Once you've inhaled fully, hold your breath for four seconds. Be comfortable, and don't strain yourself.

- **Exhale (4 seconds):** Slowly exhale through your mouth for a count of four seconds. Release the air completely from your lungs.

- **Hold (4 seconds):** After exhaling, hold your breath again for another four seconds before starting the cycle again.

- **Repeat** for as long as you need to feel calm.

The Workout Plan

This 28-day chair yoga program incorporates warm-ups and balance training first. Then, we focus on a holistic workout program that targets your entire body using cardio training, flexibility training, and strength training.

DAY	EXERCISE	DAY	EXERCISE
1	Group 1 and 2	15	Group 1 and 2
2	Group 1 and 2	16	Group 1 and 2
3	Group 1 and 3	17	Group 1, 2, 3
4	Group 1 and 3	18	Group 1, 2, 4
5	Group 1, 2, 3	19	Group 1, 2, 4
6	Break day	20	Break day
7	Group 1 and 2	21	Group 1 and 2
8	Group 1, 2, 3	22	Group 1, 2, 3
9	Group 1, 2, 3	23	All exercises
10	Group 1, 2, 4	24	All exercises
11	Group 1, 2, 4	25	All exercises
12	Group 1, 2, 4	26	All exercises
13	Break day	27	Break day
14	Group 1 and 2	28	All exercises

Gentle recovery version, if you're mobility-limited or going through rehabilitation:

- Start with group 1 for the first 1–7 days.

- Do group 1 and 2 for days 7–14.

- Do group 1, 2, and 4 for days 15–21.

- Do group 1 and 3 for days 21–28.

BALANCE EXERCISES

Every time you start a workout session, begin with these balance awareness exercises.

This is super important, especially if you are a senior. Please don't skip this.

Without proper balance awareness, we risk injury, doing the exercises incorrectly, and using bad form. This negates all the work you're putting in!

In addition, doing these balance exercises over time will also help you totally reshape the way you stand, move, and do everything.

You will feel lighter and more free instead of heavy and slow. Maybe pain in certain areas due to repetitive use and misuse will go away. Maybe your movements set feelings free, and you're aware of bad habits and correct them right away. Maybe life starts to flow again.

Try it out and go through this section every time you exercise.

Balance Check

Without stability, bad form can cause injuries and repetitive stress to your whole body. That's why we want to perform all exercises in a stable manner. As you gain stability, everything you do will feel more balanced. We'll call this "balance awareness."

The first step in balance awareness is your feet.

BALANCE CHECK INSTRUCTIONS

1   Stand straight in front of a mirror facing the wall.

2   Feel the alignment of both your feet. Are they properly aligned, or is one foot in front of the other? Are your toes pointed forward with a slight outward tilt? This is the natural alignment of the feet:

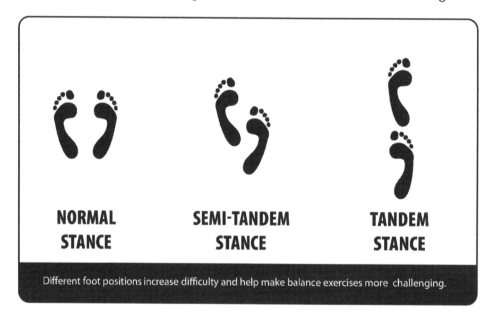

Different foot positions increase difficulty and help make balance exercises more challenging.

3   Now, feel the weight of your body on your feet. Where is the point of center? Is it toward your toes? Or are you always "on your heels?" Or always "tip-toeing" around? The center of weight should be toward the center of your foot, straight down from the ankles.

4   Stop here, take a breath, and feel your weight distribution—it should be balanced fifty-fifty on both feet. Imagine your spine passing down toward your knees and down to your ankles. The image below shows all the alignments you can build awareness around: the head controlled by the neck, the shoulders, the core and hips, your knees, and your feet.

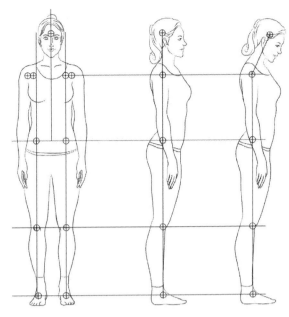

5   Use a mirror and look directly at your alignment from head to toe. Turn sideways and look now. How does your body feel? With your face forward, feel the weight distribution on your feet. Take three breaths here and just feel your body. Imagine a smooth line that goes from the top of your head down your spine and through your feet into the ground. Here are some examples of common dysfunctions:

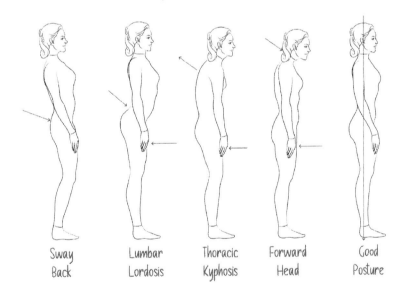

| Sway Back | Lumbar Lordosis | Thoracic Kyphosis | Forward Head | Good Posture |

Don't worry about getting it 100 percent right. Just being aware of this will increase your ability to correct any postural issues over time. This exercise trains your mind to become aware of your body's alignment as you go about your day.

Alexander Technique (Using a Chair)

The Alexander technique is a method that focuses on improving posture, movement, and overall physical coordination. Developed by F. Matthias Alexander in the 1890s, it is often used to alleviate chronic pain, improve posture, and enhance body awareness.

In this exercise, we're going to use the chair for balance as I help you find the right posture.

Many people are unaware that they have bad posture, which, over time, leads to limited mobility, pain, and other health problems.

SITTING INSTRUCTIONS

1   Using the chair as support if you feel unbalanced, feel your head, spine, and legs as you sit down. Do you feel like your whole body is aligned, or is there an uneven distribution of weight?

2   Now, try sitting down. Does your sitting down look more like the image on the left or the right below?

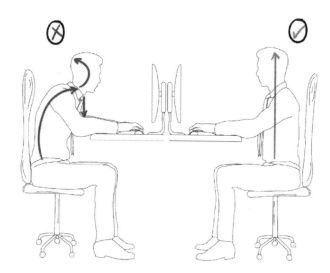

3   Try standing and sitting down three times. Each time, build awareness of how your body is moving. You may even do it in front of a bedroom mirror and watch your posture carefully.

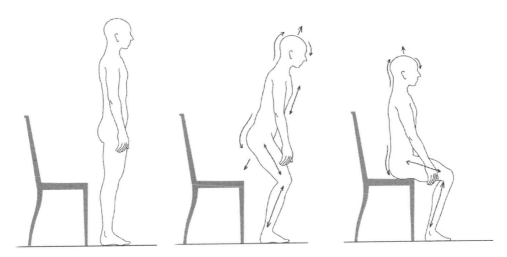

4   Now, let's try sitting down using these instructions. To sit down in a chair, we lower the trunk so that the bottom part of the pelvis or your "sit bones" can rest on the chair. Note: Your sit bones are the two bony prominences at the bottom of the pelvis that you can feel when you sit down.

5   Bend the hips, knees, and ankles so your hips feel like they are moving backward.

6   Lower your hips to the chair by flexing further, bringing your sit bones into contact with the chair, with the weight of the hips still mainly over the feet.

7   Once the sit bones are on the chair, straighten your spine so that the weight of your pelvic area is directly over the sit bones and you are sitting fully upright.

Notice how this feels compared to how you usually sit.

Alexander Technique (Standing)

Now, stand up next to the chair and explore your standing posture. Don't worry. The chair is there to support you if you lose balance or need a rest.

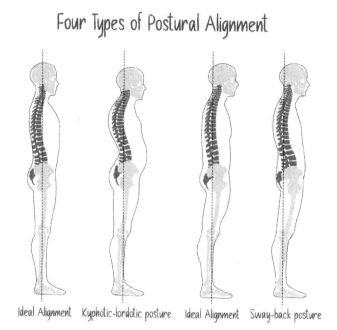

Four Types of Postural Alignment

Ideal Alignment   Kyphotic-lordotic posture   Ideal Alignment   Sway-back posture

The following standing instructions are from my mentor, a 24-year master of the Alexander technique on how to stand.

STANDING INSTRUCTIONS

Standing up straight, do the following steps:

A. The first step is "Inhibition."

Pausing. Before each movement, as well as before "directing," pause. Inhibit your tendency to react immediately to your habitual unnecessary tensions.

B. The Five Directions

1. Neck free

2. Head forward and up

3. Back lengthening and widening

4. Upper arms away from each other

5. Knees forward and away from each other

Or, simply by using intention, your body will auto-respond:

1. "I choose to allow my neck to release," or "I choose to allow my neck to soften," or "to be free" or "to unlock."

2. "I choose to allow my head to release forward and upward," or "I choose to allow an inner nodding of my head."

3. "I choose to allow my back to lengthen and widen, springing from my feet through the top of my head and expanding."

4. "I choose to allow the upper parts of my arms to go away from each other."

5. "I choose to allow my knees to go forward away from my hip joints and away from each other."

Here is how you practice the first two directions:

1) "I want" (or "I choose") to allow my neck to release."

With that intention, you ask the suboccipital muscles to unclench.

(So that my head can go forward and up.)

2) "I want" (or "I choose") to allow my head to release forward and up."

I want my head to be free to release into a nod and away from my feet.

In short: **Neck free, head forward and up.**

Remember to use intention, not "doing."

This practice will help you:

- Develop your body awareness and ability to be in the present moment.

- Make you aware of excess tension in your suboccipital area and consequently of tensions in your whole body.

- Diminish the stress placed on your neck and spine.

- Release your antigravity mechanism and ease up your whole body.

- Develop your ability to help yourself to reach, at will, your optimal state of ease.

- Help you prevent injuries.

When to practice:

Start with situations in which your mind is free to focus on yourself:

- Walking from one room to the next

- Walking from your office to your car

- Hiking

- Standing in line waiting at a counter

- Standing while talking on the phone

- Sitting while being on hold on the phone

For example, next time, notice how you use your phone, and if you're reading the Kindle version of this book, this is a good opportunity to ask: Are you overextending your neck to look down? In the graphic below, the posture in the middle is less stressful for the body than the one on the right, where the neck and hand are inefficiently extended:

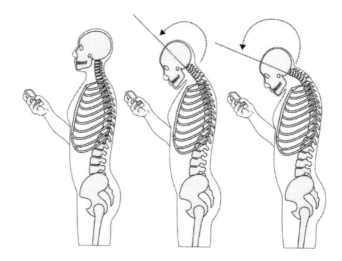

With practice, experiment in more complex situations like interacting with others or during strenuous activities involving physical effort, such as bending or lifting.

Warning: Do not "try" to make anything happen. Avoid engaging muscles in the attempt to achieve a "good" position of your head. Use the power of your intention to allow a release to happen.

Whatever position your head is in (including tilting your head backward in order to look up), you need an attitude of readiness to nod a "yes" (the "forward" direction) while you hold an intention for your head to rise upward, away from the floor.

(The "up" direction becomes "outward" direction if your body is not vertical as in lying down or bending from standing to sitting. It goes away from the base of your spine in any position.)

These first two directions are simple yet require repeated practice to identify, stop, and prevent the habits caused by a lifetime of challenges.

The next three directions integrating the whole body will be:

I want to allow my whole body to expand from my feet or my sit bones.

I want to allow my knees to go forward and away from each other.

I want to allow my shoulders to move away from each other.

Alexander used to say about the five directions: "One after the other, all at the same time." The first two directions make it possible for the whole body to expand, and at the same time, you need to be grounded for the head to be totally free to release forward and up.

I highly recommend that if you sense you have a serious postural issue, seek out a licensed Alexander technique teacher and have them guide you for a few sessions. You can find a full official list at alexandertechnique.com. Once you have "felt" the proper posture from a great teacher, return to this book to continue to the exercises.

Once you "feel" what correct posture is like, you'll want to achieve that state of freedom again and again, which is the greatest motivator.

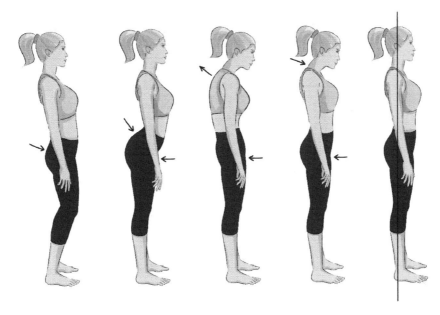

For me, when I was in constant chronic pain, after an adjustment or guidance from my Alexander technique teacher, I would always be pain-free for a few hours. Let's just say pain is a great motivator to learn!

This exercise is optional; it usually takes about ten minutes. But if you do it consistently, it will continue to improve your posture and make it into an unconscious habit. People may even start complimenting you on your posture and the way you move!

You can find great books on the Alexander technique on Amazon, but if this chapter interests you, I highly recommend finding a certified teacher and FEEL the difference in your body. In the US, that's https://www.amsatonline.org/. All the legit certified instructors require the standard 1,600 hours of training over three years!

The Monkey

This is an Alexander technique designed to build spinal awareness.

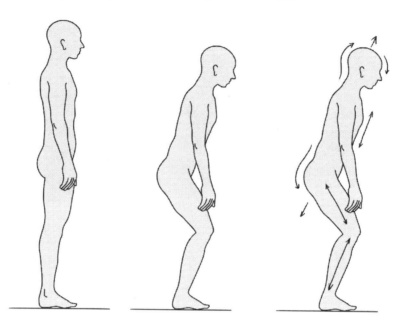

THE MONKEY INSTRUCTIONS

1 You're in a standing position. Come to your full height by allowing your neck to release to let your head go forward and up and your back to lengthen.

2 Now, think of releasing your buttocks muscles outward and downward as you bend your knees.

3 As your butt draws down and its muscles let go, think of releasing the front of your hip joints, behind your knees, and the front of your ankles. I think of this as my head leading the spine to lengthen my lower legs.

4 Allow your knees to release from your lower back, so now you're bending a bit forward but still with a straight spine. This should give you much more freedom and release in your thighs, and you will feel strength in your lower back and pelvic area. Basically, you're lengthening your back while bending your knees. This is great for lower back pain. Hang out here for a few seconds.

5 Using your leg muscles and hip muscles, push yourself back to standing. Try doing three monkeys slowly with full body awareness.

The Sky Reach

Oftentimes, prolonged body misalignment creates shortening of the muscles in the body. This creates postural dysfunctions leading to hip and back pain, shoulder pain, and head and neck pain. The inefficiencies of movement over time add unnecessary stress to your muscles and joints.

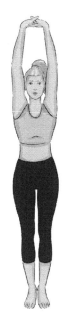

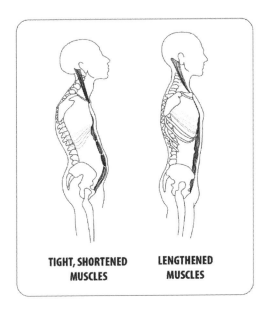

TIGHT, SHORTENED MUSCLES   **LENGTHENED MUSCLES**

We are going to do a stretch that lengthens your whole body. It's called a torso stretch in yoga, except we're going to do this with the awareness of the whole spine.

1   Standing straight, raise your hands upward.

2   Interlock your fingers, and now see how far up you can go.

3   Go as far as you can; on tiptoe is fine as you can reach further.

4   Tilt your head upward and a little backward, and stretch as far as you can. Stay here for five breaths.

5   Now release your hands and return to a normal standing position.

6   Repeat this three times.

Tips:

• Be aware of your spine alignment as you do this.

• Don't lock your knees. Keep them slightly bent and fluid.

Hip Circles

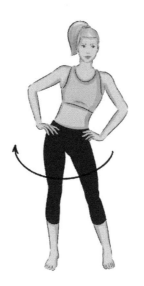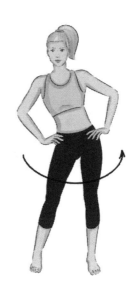

1 Stand with your feet hip-width apart and place your hands on your hips.

2 Rotate your hips outward (clockwise), keeping the upper body stable. Circle as far as you can while maintaining stability. Perform 10 circles.

3 Now rotate your hips inward (anticlockwise), keeping the upper body stable. Circle as far as you can while maintaining stability. Perform 10 circles.

Tips:

- Breathe steadily throughout the exercise.

- When doing this, feel your hips align with the spine. Do they feel intact or out of place? This is a great exercise to help you sense any posture issues with your hips.

WARM-UP EXERCISES

A proper warm-up gently activates your muscles. It gets the blood flowing and improves your joint lubrication. All this prevents potential injuries.

When I first started, I thought warm-ups were for "weak" people and that I would just "skip to the good part." Not good. I got injured, and nowadays, I always warm up.

Think of these warm-ups as a fun game! They are easy, and they feel great.

Seated Chest Claps

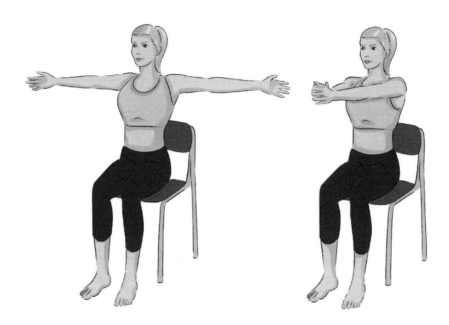

1 Sit down on a chair or on the ground with your back straight and chest up.

2 Place your hands outward with your feet comfortably apart.

3 Bring your hands together in front of your chest, then return to the starting position.

4 Go at your own pace. Speed up for faster cardio and slow down for more control. Experiment with what feels good to you.

5 Perform fifteen chest claps, keeping your core engaged.

Tips:

- Try doing this super-slow at first to get the proper form and breathing right.

- After you have the movement down, try going faster to see if you can get a sweat going. This super-fun movement is enjoyable first thing in the morning.

Chair Spinal Twist

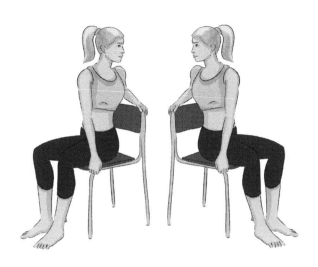

2 Place your arm on the backrest of the chair and, as you lengthen your spine, turn backward as far as you comfortably can.

3 Now return to center and turn to the other side.

4 Do 20 reps of 10 on each side.

> **Tips:**
>
> Don't sacrifice the turn distance for bad form or by twisting and tightening your core or your spine. Instead, gain length by visualizing extending your spine.

1 Sit down on a chair or on the ground with your back straight and your chest up.

Chair Side Stretch

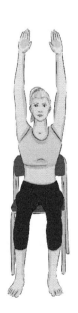 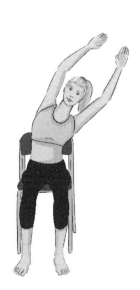

1 Sit up straight on a chair with your feet flat on the floor and your hands raised high up in the air.

2 Take a few breaths and lengthen your spine. As you do, lean to the right with your hands leading.

3 Now return to center and turn to the other side.

4 Perform twenty reps of ten on each side.

> **Tips:**
>
> Don't sacrifice the leaning distance by tightening muscles. Gain mobility by lengthening your muscles.

Cobra Pose Chair

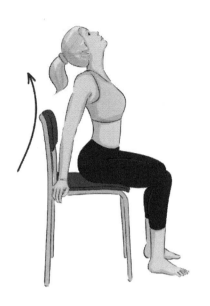

1   Sit halfway to the edge and straight up on a chair with your feet flat on the floor. Place your hands behind you firmly on the seat.

2   As you inhale, lengthen your spine and lift your chest. Arch your back and tilt your head upward and backward as far as you can.

3   As you exhale, slowly return to a normal sitting position.

4   Do ten reps.

Tips:

Don't sit too close to the edge as it's dangerous. Find the center and scoot just enough to place your hands on the chair firmly.

Chair Downward Stretch

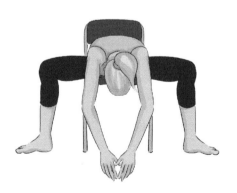

1   Sit up straight on a chair with your legs as widely extended as possible.

2   Inhale a deep breath. As you exhale, bend forward with your hands as far down as you can.

3   Repeat five times. Each time you extend down, try to go a little further.

Tips:

- Avoid sitting or sitting too close to the chair's edge.

- If you're super-flexible and can touch the ground, see if you can bring your elbows to the ground.

Chair Arm Circle

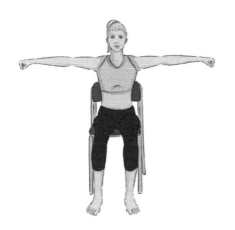 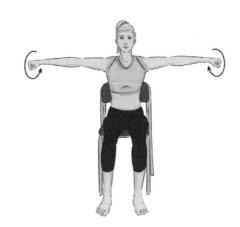

1 Sit up straight on a chair with your feet flat on the floor.

2 Extend your arms straight out to the sides, parallel to the floor.

3 Begin making small circular motions with your arms, like you're drawing circles with your hands. You can use an open-handed palm or your fists.

4 Continue the circular motions for ten seconds.

5 Now, go in the other direction for ten seconds.

Tips:

• Maintain slow and controlled movements to avoid straining your shoulders.

• Gradually increase the size of the circles as you feel comfortable.

CARDIO EXERCISES

There are many benefits to cardiovascular exercise, from improved metabolism to improved lung capacity and improved sleep... the list goes on.

If you've heard the term "Yoga Body," it's because the following exercises not only use cardio to burn calories, they also strengthen and tone your muscle groups at the same time so you end up looking amazing.

Our main goal is not weight loss. It's just a byproduct of this form of exercise. You see... we are using low-impact exercises designed to strengthen muscles, improve postural alignment, and enhance flexibility.

So not only will you lose weight if you do these exercises consistently while having a balanced diet... you'll feel stronger, more flexible, and move with a more aligned posture. Is that motivating enough for you?

Let's get started!

Chair Leg Extension

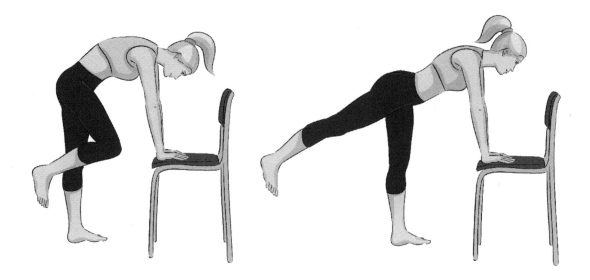

1 Place your hands on the sides of the chair seat for stability.

2 Lift one leg off the ground, then extend it fully behind you.

3 Hold your leg extended for three seconds.

4 Now, return your leg back to the starting position slowly. It's still lifted from the ground.

5 Repeat this ten times.

6 Change legs and repeat this extension ten times.

7 Breathe naturally as you perform the leg extensions.

Tips:

• Keep your back straight, engage your core, and maintain control throughout the exercise.

• You can speed up or increase reps as you become more familiar with this exercise.

The Sparrow

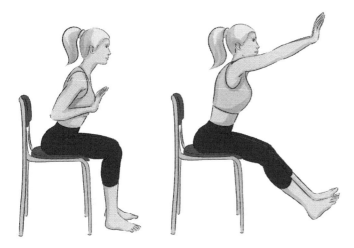

1 Sit in a chair leaning forward with your hands in front of your chest.

2 Extend your hands upward and your feet forward at the same time at about a 45-degree angle upward and downward, respectively.

3 Come back to the original position and repeat fifteen times.

Tips:

Keep your spine straight as you do this.

Sitting Duck Pose

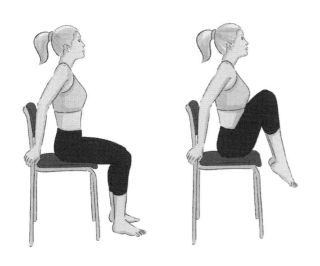

1 Begin by sitting and placing your hands on the back of the chair for stability.

2 As you exhale, bend your knees and lift your legs. Keep your weight on your sit bones.

3 Hold for up to three seconds. Try to breathe and maintain balance.

4 Return your feet to the ground.

5 Repeat this ten times.

Tips:

You can increase the hold for up to five seconds as you get stronger.

Torso Twist

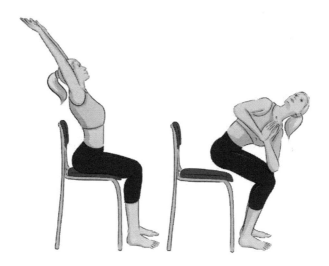

1. Sit upright in a sturdy chair with your feet flat on the ground.

2. Reach upward and backward with your hands, arching your arms for a good stretch.

3. Bring your arms downward all the way and turn to the right, placing your elbow between or close to your knees. Hold here for three seconds as you take deep breaths.

4. Reach upward again for a good stretch, and this time, come down, turning left as you place your elbows between or close to your knees.

5. Repeat the movement, switching from left to right and again up to a total of ten times (five on each side).

Tips:

Move on the exhale for a burst of energy. You can also move on the inhale and exhale to use your breath to guide your movements.

Chair Warrior Pose

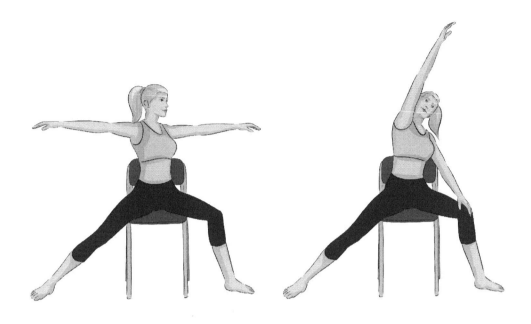

1. Start in a sitting position with your feet three to four feet apart with the chair in the middle as a stabilizer.

2. Turn your left foot out while your right foot straightens outward.

3. Extend your arms out to the sides.

4. Bend your left knee to a 90-degree angle while keeping your right leg straight.

5. Keep your torso facing forward and gaze over your left hand. Hold the warrior pose here for five seconds.

6. Now, move your right hand upward and to the left as far as you comfortably can. Hold for five seconds.

7. Do this for five reps.

8. Now repeat this for the other side (right foot 90-degree angle, left foot straight).

Tips:

As you get stronger, you can do this without the chair.

Dancer Pose

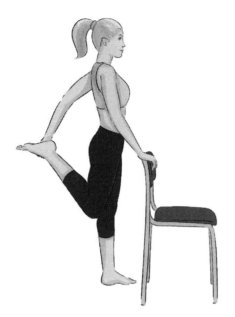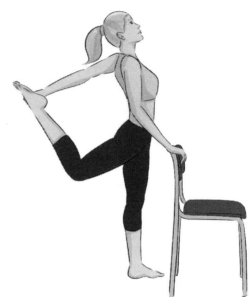

1 Stand behind the chair and use one hand to stabilize yourself.

2 Lift your right foot backward and hold it with your left hand.

3 Extend your legs and spine and lift your leg even further upward and backward. Hold for five seconds, then release.

4 Repeat five times.

5 Now do this for the other side (left foot backward, holding it with your right hand).

6 Repeat five times.

Tips:

As you gain increased balance, you can do this without holding onto the chair. You can still stand close to the chair for support in case you lose balance.

Sitting Jacks

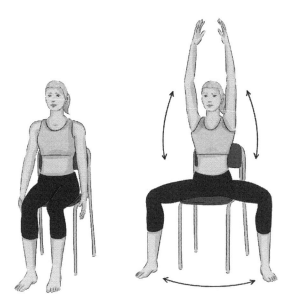

1. Sit on a chair with your feet flat on the floor and your back straight.

2. Start with your feet together and your arms at your sides.

3. In one fluid motion, jump your feet apart and raise your arms overhead, just like a traditional jumping jack, but while remaining seated.

4. Return to the starting position with your feet together and your arms at your sides.

5. Repeat this up to fifteen times. Try to maintain a steady rhythm.

Tips:

- You can increase the speed and intensity of this for more cardio and slow it down for more flexibility and control.

- You can increase the reps to thirty as you gain strength and endurance.

FLEXIBILITY EXERCISES

In Pilates as well as yoga...

Control = Flexibility + Strength

In this section, we are not doing rapid, high-repetition sets but rather performing slower, precise movements with full muscular control. Remember the tai chi and Pilates concepts mentioned earlier? In fact, some Pilates instructors ban the use of the word "exercise" and instead use the word "movement" in their books and trainings.

Why is this important? Because with slow, controlled movements, we are working out our fast-twitch muscle fibers (type II) and slow-twitch muscle fibers (type I) for maximum gains. We also reduce the risk of injury while doing so.

Chair Eagle

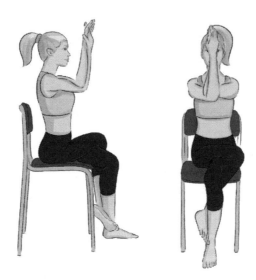

1   Sit on a chair with your feet flat on the floor and your back straight.

2   Lift your right leg and cross it over your left thigh as if you were sitting cross-legged.

3   If possible, tuck your right foot behind your left calf for a deeper stretch.

4   Cross your arms in front of your chest with your right arm under your left.

5   Bend your elbows and bring your palms together if you can. If not, simply touch your opposite shoulders with your hands.

6   Sit up straight and engage your core.

7   Hold the chair eagle pose for fifteen seconds, feeling a stretch in your upper back and hips.

8   Release and repeat on the other side by lifting your left leg and crossing it over your right thigh with your left arm under your right. Hold for fifteen seconds.

9   Repeat this five times on each side.

> **Tips:**
>
> You can start with your legs only and work on your focus and form before moving onto your arms.

Cat Stretch & Breathwork

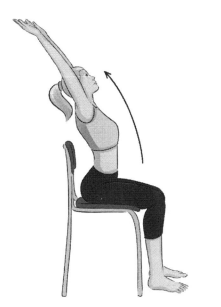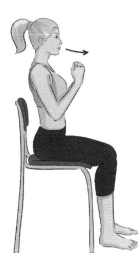

1 Sit on a chair with your feet flat on the ground and your back straight.

2 Interlace your fingers and take three deep breaths.

3 Extend your arms upward and backward with your palms open, lengthening your spine. Gently arch your back and look up if it's comfortable for your neck.

4 Hold this stretch for fifteen seconds.

5 Return to an upright, seated position with fingers crossed and take three deep breaths.

6 Repeat this three times, focusing on your breath and maintaining good posture.

Tips:

Remember your breathwork from the first few chapters? This is a great movement to practice the relaxing breath (the 4-7-8 technique).

Heel Raises

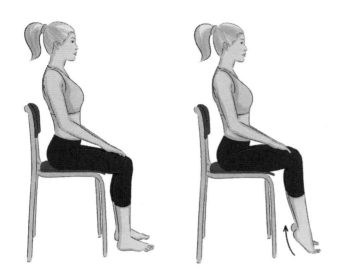

1. Sit on a chair with your feet flat on the floor and your back straight.

2. Place your hands on your thighs for stability.

3. Slowly lift your heels off the ground, raising them as high as you comfortably can.

4. Hold the raised position for a second or two.

5. Lower your heels back to the floor.

6. Repeat this motion fifteen times or up to twenty at a level that's comfortable for you.

Tips:

Remember to keep your back straight.

Floor Leg Raise

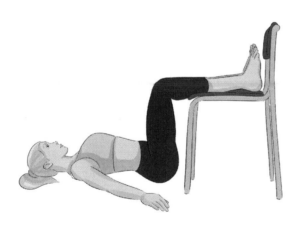

1. Lie down on a mat or the floor with your legs at a 90-degree angle on the chair.

2. Place your arms at your sides, palms facing up.

3. Relax and breathe deeply, holding the pose for thirty seconds. Sometimes, I stay here for up to a minute.

Tips:

You can raise your hands to the sides fully extended like a cross. This is also found in the Egoscue method. It realigns the hips and legs.

Upward Hand Stretch

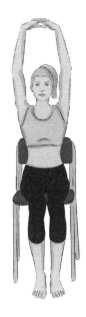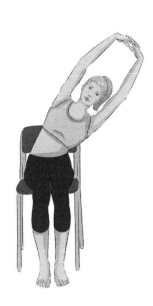

1   Sit on a chair with your back straight and your feet flat on the floor.

2   Inhale deeply as you extend both arms overhead, reaching for the sky.

3   Keep your palms facing upward and your fingers extended. Stretch your entire upper body, lengthening your spine. Feel the stretch from your fingertips to your shoulders.

4   Now move your arms to the right for five seconds; hold here, and take two deep breaths.

5   Now repeat on the left side.

6   To exit, gently lower your arms back to your thighs.

Tips:

· Remember to keep your head looking forward and your spine straight.

· You can repeat the stretch as needed to relieve upper body tension and improve posture while seated.

Chair Leg Raise

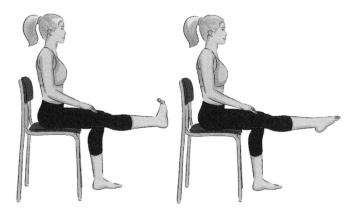

3 Slowly lift one leg straight out in front of you with your toes pointed upward. Now, point them forward parallel to the floor.

4 Gently lower your leg back to the floor.

5 Repeat the motion five times.

6 Repeat the leg raise on the other side.

Tips:

You can place your hands on the sides of the chair or hold the armrests for support.

1 Sit on a chair with your back straight and your feet flat on the floor.

2 Engage your core muscles to stabilize your body.

Chair Cat-Cow

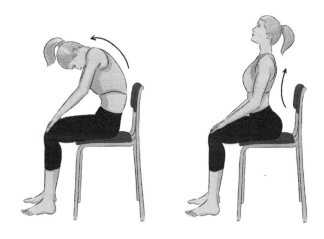

4 As you exhale, round your back, tuck your chin to your chest, and draw your navel in (cat pose).

5 Continue to flow between cow and cat poses with your breath, inhaling for the cow and exhaling for the cat.

6 Perform this gentle movement for ten reps, feeling the stretch and release in your spine.

1 Sit on a chair with your feet flat on the floor and your back straight.

2 Place your hands on your knees or thighs.

3 Inhale and arch your back, lifting your chest (cow pose).

Tips:

• You can place your hands on the sides of the chair or hold the armrests for support.

• Keep your movements smooth and controlled, focusing on your breath and the sensations in your back.

Hand Stretch

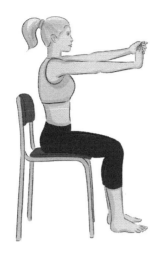 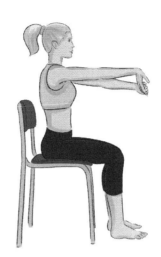

1   Sit or stand with your back straight.

2   Extend your right arm in front of you at shoulder height, palm facing outward.

3   With your left hand, gently grasp your right fingers or thumb.

4   Apply gentle pressure to stretch your fingers back toward your body.

5   Hold the stretch for fifteen seconds, feeling a gentle pull in your hand and fingers.

6   Switch to your left hand and repeat the stretch.

7   You can also stretch your fingers individually by gently pulling them backward.

Tips:

•   Perform the stretch as needed to relieve hand tension and improve hand flexibility.

•   You can do this anytime, even while standing up.

•   Keep your head facing forward and your spine aligned when doing this.

Chair Leg Kicks

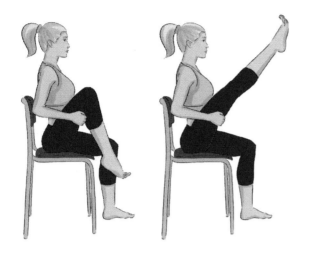

2   Place both hands below one of your thighs and lift your thigh.

3   Now extend your feet upward. It's okay if you can't extend your leg completely straight. Just go as far as you comfortably can.

4   Release your leg and return to position 2 (both hands below the thigh).

5   Do seven reps.

6   Now repeat for the other leg.

Tips:

Try to keep your toes straight when your feet are off the floor.

1   Sit on a chair with your feet flat on the floor, your back straight, and your hands on your thighs for stability.

Seated Knee Stretch

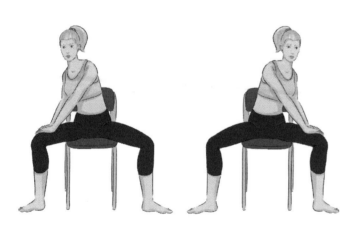

3   Hold for three seconds.

4   Now, turn and hold the other knee with your hands. Hold for three seconds.

5   Repeat this for a total of five times on each knee.

Tips:

Keep your head up and your spine aligned. Gain length by extending, not tightening, muscles

1   Sit comfortably on the chair and spread your legs as much as possible.

2   Place both hands on one knee and lean slightly forward. The turn comes from the torso, not the hips.

Chair Half Warrior Pose

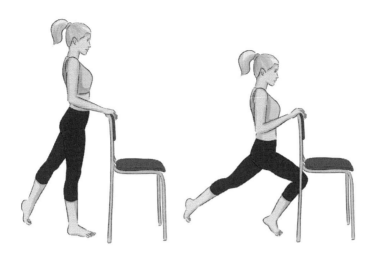

1 Begin in a standing position behind the chair.

2 Step your left foot back about three to four feet. As you do, bend your right knee and extend your left leg backward as far as you comfortably can.

3 Hold here for ten seconds. You can even push a little bit to see if you can go further. Use the chair for stability so you can push harder and further.

4 To exit the pose, step your back foot forward to the starting position.

5 Repeat the pose on the other side by stepping your right foot back and bending your left knee.

6 Repeat this exercise five times on each side.

Tips:

- As you gain more balance, you can put the chair to the side just in case you lose balance.

- You can also extend your arms toward the front and the back as in a normal warrior pose.

Standing Head Stretch

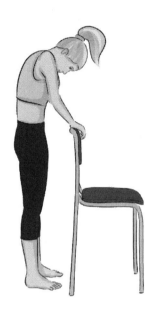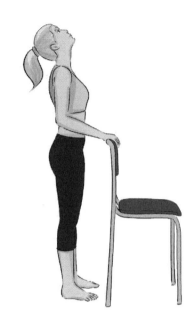

1 Stand with your back straight and your shoulders relaxed. Put your hands on the back of the chair for support.

2 Inhale deeply and, as you exhale, tilt your head downward, bringing your chin toward your chest. Hold for five seconds.

3 Now, raise your head upward and backward. Hold for five seconds.

4 Perform the downward and upward stretch for eight reps.

Tips:

• You can repeat this stretch as needed to relieve tension in your neck and shoulders. I do ten reps each morning.

• Keep your feet on the ground and your legs straight. A slight bend on the knees is fine.

Seated Stretch & Bend

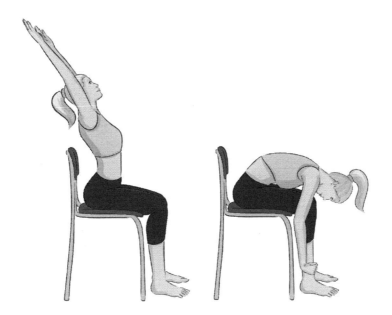

1 Sit on a chair with your back straight, your feet flat on the ground, and your hands resting on your thighs.

2 Inhale deeply and, as you exhale, raise your arms above and behind your head, reaching for the ceiling.

3 Hold the stretch for ten seconds, breathing deeply and evenly.

4 Now lean forward, bringing your chest to your knees, and go as deep as you can. Hold for ten seconds.

5 Repeat the above eight times.

Tips:

- You can hold your ankles when you go downward for stability.

- You can repeat both upward and downward stretches as needed to relieve tension and promote flexibility while sitting.

Seated Head & Arm Stretch

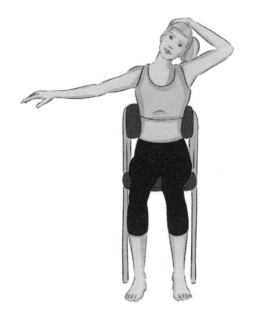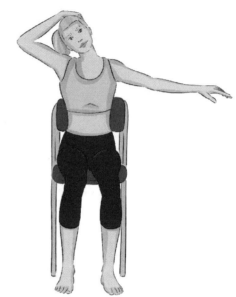

1 Sit on a chair with your feet flat on the ground and your back straight.

2 Place your right hand on your left ear and gently guide your head to the right, bringing your right ear toward your right shoulder.

3 Hold the head tilt for ten to fifteen seconds, feeling a gentle stretch along the left side of your neck.

4 Release your head and return it to an upright position.

5 Repeat this for the other side.

6 Perform these stretches as needed to relieve neck and arm tension and improve flexibility. I do five stretches each on the left and right side for a total of ten reps.

Tips:

- Be careful not to use too much force with your hand moving your head. Only go as far as comfortable.

- If you feel any pain at all, stop immediately. Some people have tension around the sternocleidomastoid (SCM) muscle and the levator scapulae muscle. In this case, consider releasing the trigger points first.

Seated Half Moon Pose

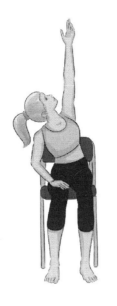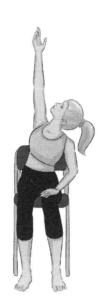

1 Sit on the chair with your legs in front of you.

2 Place your right hand on your lap. Inhale and lift your left arm overhead, stretching it toward the right side.

3 Exhale and extend your left hand upward.

4 Hold the pose for ten seconds, feeling a stretch along your left side.

5 Inhale and return to an upright seated position.

6 Repeat the stretch on the other side, placing your left hand on your lap and reaching your right arm overhead.

7 Perform these stretches as needed to improve flexibility and balance. I do five reps on each side for a total of ten.

Tips:

You can extend your resting hand toward the floor instead of your lap for a deeper stretch.

Chair Squat

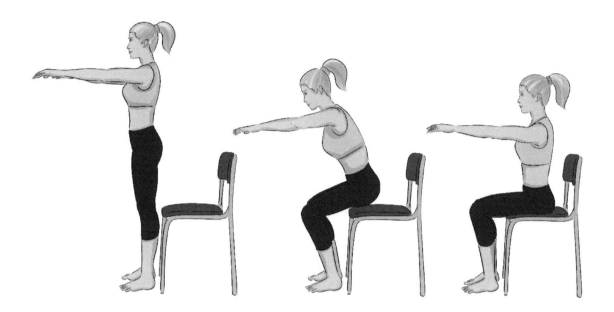

1 Sit on the edge of a sturdy chair with your feet flat on the ground, hip-width apart. Keep your back straight, your shoulders relaxed, and your arms by your sides.

2 As you exhale and engage your leg muscles, lift your hips off the chair.

3 Use your leg muscles to push through your heels to rise to a standing position. Hold the standing position for three seconds, ensuring your knees are not locked.

4 On your exhale, gently lower yourself back down to the chair.

5 Repeat the chair squat ten times, maintaining a controlled and smooth motion.

6 Focus on your breath and keep your core engaged to maintain balance.

Tips:

Think of your spine as aligned at all times as you move from a sitting to a standing position. Remember your posture training in exercises 1–3 and the Alexander technique.

Next Steps

"Take care of your body. It's the only place you have to live."
— Jim Rohn

Once you get into the habit of these movements, you won't want to stop. Use the 28-Day Challenge program to stay motivated and on track. After a while... doing regular chair yoga exercises will make you feel more flexible, stronger, toned, and more vibrant in every way. After about eight weeks, this will become a habit for the rest of your life.

I know that some of you will want to continue on to more advanced exercises, so before we say goodbye, let me direct you to our exclusive free book on pelvic floor Kegels exercise at wallpilates.org as taught by Tim Sawyer, a leading physical therapist who worked with Dr. Anderson and Dr. Wise at the Stanford University Medical Center[*].

You can also check out our other exercise books here on Amazon.

You can also scan the following to get your free bonus:

---

[*]   Authors of *A Headache in the Pelvis: A New Understanding and Treatment for Chronic Pelvic Pain Syndromes*.

Thank You

My name is Luna, and it has been my pleasure to serve you.

You could have picked from dozens of other books, but you took a chance and chose this one.

So, thank you for investing in yourself and making it to the end!

Before we say goodbye, one question: If you enjoyed this book, would you consider leaving a review? A review is the easiest and best way to support the work of independent authors like me. Your feedback will help us continue writing the types of books that will help you and others in the journey to good health.

How to leave a review in fifteen seconds:

Chair Yoga And Wall Pilates Book

mybook.to/wallpilatesforseniors

Pilates is a safe, effective, and beautiful movement technique that helps seniors improve their lives. From recovering from chronic pain to staying in shape as we age to feeling stronger and healthier... it adds value no matter which stage of life you're in right now.

As you work on these exercises, by the fifth or sixth session, you will start to feel more aligned in your posture and feel like you're standing taller.

By the tenth session, you won't want to stop.

By the twentieth session, it will become a habit.

This technique invented by Joseph Pilates literally gave me my life back after a car accident. I hope now, with the exercises in this book, you can enjoy these all the benefits Pilates has to offer you from the comfort of your own home. I'd like to end with a quote that you read at the start of this book from Joseph Pilates himself:

"In 10 sessions, you'll feel the difference. In 20, you'll see the difference. And in 30, you'll be on your way to having a whole new body."

– Joseph Pilates[*]

If you haven't started yet, what are you waiting for? Try out these movements for yourself and feel the truth in your body.

To your happiness and health,

— Luna Light

---

[*]   Pilates and Miller. Return to Life through Contrology.

Additional Resources

Luna Light's author page on Amazon:

https://www.amazon.com/stores/Luna-Light/author

Citations

Cover Image Source: Free license from Freepik.com and copyrighted images from our illustrators at Luna Light publishing.

Images used in this book: Free license from Freepik.com

Disclosures

Some of the links provided in this book are affiliate links, which help you jump to the exact URL of the resource you're looking for at no additional cost to you.

The Legal Stuff

Assumption of Risk: By reading/using this book, the User/Reader acknowledges that physical exercise involves inherent risks and hazards. By choosing to follow or participate in any exercise regimen, instruction, or advice detailed in the Book, the User expressly and voluntarily assumes all risks associated with such activities, recognizing that they may result in injury, illness, death, and/or damage to personal property.

Waiver: By reading this book/guide, the User hereby waives, releases, and forever discharges the author, publisher, and all related parties from any and all claims, liabilities, actions, suits, demands, costs, losses, damages, attorney's fees, and expenses, whether known or unknown, foreseen, or unforeseen that arise out of or relate to the User's/Reader's use of or reliance on the Book/Workout Guide.

"In 10 sessions, you'll feel the difference. In 20, you'll see the difference. And in 30, you'll be on your way to having a whole new body."*
– Joseph Pilates

---

*   Joseph H. Pilates and William J. Miller. *Return to Life through Contrology,* (Mockingbird Press, 2021).

Magic in Movement as We Age

"The body is like a piano, and happiness is like music. It is needful to have the instrument in good order."
– Henry Ward Beecher

After the age of fifty, the human body experiences many changes that lead to weight gain, muscle loss, and poor posture. Hormone changes, loss of bone density, and muscle atrophy are just some of the reasons. Without a proper plan, it's an easy path to limited mobility and having our bodies feel sluggish and tired all the time.

Yet, for every case of limited mobility and dwindling health, there are 50, 60, 70, and 80+ year-olds who are vibrant, full of energy, and have freedom in their movements. For example, have you ever walked by a group of elders doing tai chi in the morning?

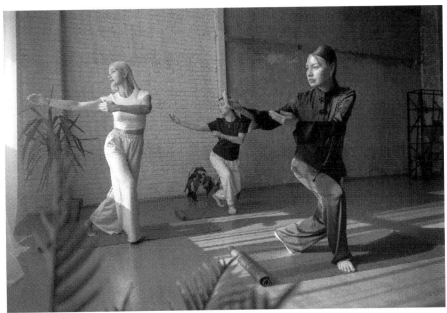

One of the main philosophies in tai chi is that instead of fighting against "it" (life, your muscles, your body limitations), we instead adapt and evolve with it. Tai chi movements follow the breath and use the natural flow of chi to guide slow, comfortable movements.

Have you ever seen a Pilates class in action?

In *Caged Lion*, John Howard Steel talks about "Pilates [as] a system of coordinated movement, concentration, and breathing that fully absorbs the actor in what he or she is doing, adds grace and efficiency to daily life, relieves stress, increases circulation, augments self-esteem, becomes a habit, and most importantly is fun to do.'"

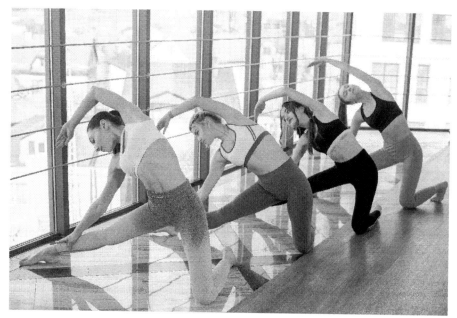

Both Pilates and tai chi emphasize the presence and accuracy of slow moments. By going slow, we're actually getting gains faster by concentrating all the muscles in the movements.

The philosophy of both movements also allows us to accept and adapt to aging instead of constantly fighting against it and resisting the natural aging process.

The practical aspects of tai chi and Pilates ensure that we don't get injured as we get our bodies strong again.

So...as you do the following exercises, I invite you to think about the philosophy of slow, controlled movements guided by your breath and the natural energy flow of your body.

Let's get into it!

*   John Howard Steel. *Caged Lion: Joseph Pilates & His Legacy* (p. 178). Last Leaf Press. Kindle Edition.

Why Wall Pilates for Seniors?

"Change happens through movement, and movement heals."
– Joseph Pilates[*]

Five years ago, the secrets I learned using wall Pilates after a car accident helped me get out of chronic pain. At the time, I was in so much pain I could not walk and was restricted to my bedroom, with a small floor area and a wall. Necessity forced me to discover new ways of exercising and getting my life back.

As I recovered from the pain using Pilates movements, I continued to strengthen my body, and I was surprised to find even more health benefits like the ones you'll discover in the following chapter. Although I was in an accident, doctors told me that the pain became chronic because of the wear and tear of my body as I got older. Therefore, a big part of my rehabilitation was restrengthening my muscles for functional use again. This is why I believe you can heal your body using these techniques.

Wall Pilates doesn't require complex equipment, is beginner-friendly, and is space- and cost-effective. You can do it anywhere, anytime. Even when I'm traveling without a yoga mat, I simply place a towel on the floor and begin my wonderful workout.

While yoga and regular Pilates can improve your health, wall Pilates focuses on using the resistance of the wall to build up your core strength, burn calories, and align and improve your posture. Here's how I explain the difference to prospective students:

---

[*]   Pilates and Miller. *Return to Life through Contrology*

Feature	Wall Pilates	Regular Pilates	Yoga
Equipment	Wall, Yoga Mat	Reformer, Wunda Chair, Trapeze Table, Ladder Barrel, and more...	Yoga Mat, Yoga Blocks
Cost	$40 Yoga Mat	$50-100 membership $150 per private session	$40 Yoga Mat
Level Of Difficulty	Beginner To Advanced Beginner Friendly and Senior Friendly	Intermediate to Advanced	Beginner To Advanced
Focus Of Benefits	Core strength, posture, flexibility and pain relief. The wall offers an added dimension of resistance and alignment feedback.	Core strength, coordination, and endurance	Meditation, Flexibility, balance, and mental focus, focusing on inner peace and presence

In addition, we will look to gain:

1. **More Muscle Tone:** Pushing or pulling against the wall helps to tone and strengthen various muscle groups, enhancing overall muscle definition (aka the Pilates body).

2. **Better Posture:** The wall offers immediate feedback, helping you build spinal awareness and correct postural misalignments. Over time, this can lead to better posture, which is crucial not just for aesthetics but also for reducing strain on the spine and other joints.

3. **Improved Flexibility:** By leveraging the wall, we can safely deepen the stretches because the wall can support the weight of certain body parts, allowing for extended stretch durations and a greater range of motion.

4. **Stress Reduction:** Pilates emphasizes deep breathing and focused movement. This mindfulness can help alleviate stress as attention is drawn away from external pressures and directed toward the body's movement and breath. You're so focused you literally don't have time to worry.

5. **Sexual Stamina and Flexibility:** Improved pelvic floor strength, flexibility, and increased blood flow—all benefits of working your core—can lead to enhanced sexual stamina and flexibility. A strengthened core (that includes the pelvic muscles) can heighten both control and sensation. In fact, Mr. Pilates said in his own words, "So, Contrology strengthens the body and makes it work good for sex. And sex makes people happy and healthier.**"

** Steel. *Caged Lion: Joseph Pilates & His Legacy*.

6. **Improved Mental Acuity:** The concentration required in wall Pilates requires a mindful presence and focus, which helps you improve practice shifting into focus in other areas of your life.

7. **Better Sleep:** Regular exercise has been linked to improved sleep patterns. Wall Pilates, with its emphasis on relaxation, breathing, and physical exertion, can result in deeper and more restful sleep. You can even use some of the breathing techniques in this book to prime your body for relaxation before going to bed.

Sometimes, it's hard for a beginner to see how powerful Pilates movements are, so let's illustrate all the muscles you stimulate in just one movement called "the teaser."

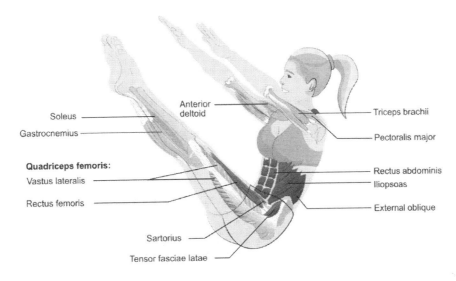

Twelve muscles, type I and II muscle fibers, small to large! Remarkable, isn't it?

In humans, type I or slow-twitch fibers are fatigue-resistant and help everyday function. For example, the soleus leg muscle (the muscle behind your lower leg) is type I.

Type II fibers, or fast oxidative glycolytic (FOG) fibers, present higher twitch speeds than type I fibers but are less fatigue-resistant. They give you a burst of energy and are involved in fast movements. For example, your biceps and triceps muscles are mostly type II.

Just know that when you exercise from this book, we will be working more of your muscles, all kinds of muscles (types I and II), and from small to large muscles, all more efficiently than any other exercise technique I know, with little to no risk of injury.

YOUR FREE GIFTS

I want to remind you that a free gift comes with your purchase of this book: the Ultimate Kegels Guide.

This guide helps you strengthen your core and improve your intimate life. Kegels are often done incorrectly, but these instructions are from Tim Sawyer, a top physical therapist who worked with doctors at Stanford University* to develop chronic pain rehabilitation programs.

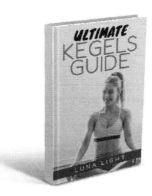

All you have to do is go to wallpilates.org to download it for free. Alternatively, scan the QR code below:

---

*   Dr. Wise and Dr. Anderson authored *A Headache in the Pelvis: A New Understanding and Treatment for Chronic Pelvic Pain Syndromes* (Harmony: 2018) and consulted Tim as the main physical therapist for their treatments.

What You Need to Start

"You don't have to be great to start, but you have to start to be great."
— Zig Ziglar

Before we begin, do a quick check for:

1. **A Sturdy Wall:** Ensure the wall you're using is solid and can withstand pressure. Avoid walls with loose plaster, as pushing or leaning against them could lead to unexpected breaks or collapses.

2. **Clear Space:** Ensure the area around the wall is free from obstacles; slippery rugs, glass, or loose items that could lead to trips or falls.

3. **Footwear and Attire:** Wear appropriate nonslip footwear if you prefer. Pilates is very effective barefoot. Comfortable, form-fitting attire can help you move freely without getting tangled or caught.

4. **Staying Hydrated:** Drink plenty of water before, during, and after your wall Pilates session to prevent muscle cramps and promote recovery. I always prepare a water bottle before a workout.

5. **Yoga Mat:** A good yoga mat can help you gain traction and make lying on the floor easier and more comfortable. This is optional but recommended.

When exercising, if you feel like you're pushing too hard... it's okay to rest and then start again slowly. Consistency is more important than "going hard."

My mentor once told me: "Being extraordinary is simply performing ordinary things consistently over a period of time."

We are going against the "go go go!" trend of most of the fitness industry.

Stop. Instead, we are going to go at our own pace. This isn't a race... there's no competition here.

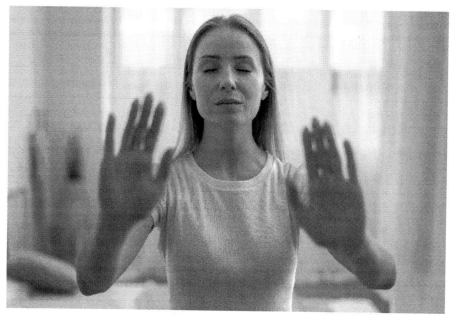

"The focus was all on the doing and not on competing, even with yourself. There were no objective goals such as do more exercises, or faster, or use more resistance. Progress was felt, not measured."

– John Howard Steel
Caged Lion: Joseph Pilates & His Legacy

How to Breathe When You Move

"Breathing is the first act of life and the last. Our very life depends on it. Since we cannot live without breathing, it is tragically deplorable to contemplate the millions and millions who have never mastered the art of correct breathing."
– Joseph Pilates[*]

There are many nuances to breathwork during Pilates. The most important thing to remember is the coordination of the breath to help the movement of your body.

When starting out, here are some safe breathing techniques you can experiment with. Different teachers teach different breathing techniques, so try a few and find the one that resonates most with you.

Inhale through the nose: Taking a deep breath in, aim to expand the ribcage out to the sides, allowing the lungs to fill up with air.

Exhale through the mouth: Purse your lips as if you're blowing out through a straw and exhale fully, engaging your core muscles and feeling the abdominal wall draw inward.

Timing with Movement

As a general rule, exhale during the effort or exertion phase of an exercise and inhale during the return or relaxation phase.

For example, when doing a Pilates teaser, you'd exhale as you lift your upper body up toward the sky and inhale as you lower it back down.

Enhancing Stretch and Range

You can use your breath to deepen stretches. Typically, inhaling prepares for the movement, and exhaling allows you to sink deeper into the stretch.

---

[*]   Pilates and Miller. *Return to Life through Contrology*

Using Breath to Expand

Sometimes I go into a lightning pose and practice breathing for ten reps. During each rep, I imagine my rib cage expanding. Then I imagine my abdomen expanding, then my upper back, then my lower back. With each breath, I see if I can expand my lungs and diaphragm in all directions. This practice has improved my breathing capacity significantly after just a few months. If you use your mouth to inhale and exhale, you can expand further with more air and then revert back to nose breathing on subsequent counts.

Pacing and Rhythm When Moving

Maintaining a steady breathing rhythm can help set the pace for your exercises. It promotes a mindful approach, preventing rushing through movements and ensuring each exercise is performed with precision.

4-7-8 Technique

The 4-7-8 technique, also known as the "relaxing breath," is a simple breathing exercise developed by Dr. Andrew Weil. It's inspired by an ancient yogic technique called *pranayama*, which involves the regulation of breath to enhance physical and mental well-being.

The 4-7-8 technique is designed to act as a natural tranquilizer for the nervous system, so it's great at the end of a workout. In fact, I use it whenever I feel rushed or stressed outside the gym.

4-7-8 Steps:

1. Inhale quietly through the nose for a count of four.

2. Hold your breath for a count of seven.

3. Exhale completely through the mouth, making a whoosh sound for a count of eight.

4. This is one breath cycle. Aim to complete this cycle for four breaths while you relax.

Box Breathing

Box breathing, also known as square breathing, is a relaxation and stress reduction technique that has been utilized in various practices, including yoga, meditation, and tactical settings in the military. The best part about this is that it's easy to remember: 4 seconds in, 4 seconds hold, 4 seconds out, 4 seconds hold.

The technique itself has deep roots in ancient practices, especially in disciplines such as yoga and meditation. These ancient practices aim to regulate and control the breath to improve physical, mental, and emotional well-being. Here are the practice instructions:

Breathing Pattern: Follow this sequence for each breath phase:

- **Inhale (4 seconds):** Breathe in slowly and deeply through your nose for a count of four seconds. Feel your lungs expanding as you do so.

- **Hold (4 seconds):** Once you've inhaled fully, hold your breath for four seconds. Be comfortable, and don't strain yourself.

- **Exhale (4 seconds):** Slowly exhale through your mouth for a count of four seconds. Release the air completely from your lungs.

- **Hold (4 seconds):** After exhaling, hold your breath again for another four seconds before starting the cycle again.

- **Repeat** for as long as you need to feel calm.

My Chronic Pain Story

Years ago, a car accident sent me to the ER at UCLA with a stabbing-like pain in my abdominal wall and pelvic floor. The doctors could not find anything wrong, but what followed were months of tests, MRIs, blood draws, CT scans, and hospital visits. Even with all that, no one could tell me what was wrong with my body or why I was in pain. I spent the next two years searching for a way to cure my chronic pain syndrome.[*]

While many things contributed to my healing, when I started doing Pilates... I immediately started feeling better. After my first few sessions, the changes I experienced in my body made me realize that there was a way to fully recover!

While everyone's body is different, and chronic pain can have overlapping and complicated causes, I discovered that my chronic pain was coming from weak muscles riddled with trigger points (TrPs). Trigger points are taut muscle bands that have been created that restrict movement and blood flow. If you feel like you have TrPs, a great place to start is Clair Davies's book **The Trigger Point Therapy Workbook.**

So, if you have muscles ridden with TrPs like I did, you must first get rid of those TrPs. But what comes later is a weak TrPs-free muscle. This is where Pilates comes in. I trained my weak muscles to get stronger with Pilates since it can work all the slow- and fast-twitch muscle fibers and regulate smaller muscles that aren't stimulated to the same extent by conventional exercises.

As I improved my precision in my Pilates exercises, the pelvic and abdominal pain slowly faded away. The origin of the pain and dysfunction—weak and TrP-ridden muscles—started to disappear.

I am now pain-free thanks to Pilates, and it continues to improve my strength, stamina, sex life, and mental well-being. I hope it can do the same for you!

---

[*]   Pain becomes "chronic" when it lasts more than six months without a proper diagnosis.

GENTLE WARM-UP ROUTINE

A proper warm-up gently activates your muscles. It gets the blood flowing and improves your joint lubrication. All this prevents potential injuries.

I know most people skip warm-ups. Don't' skip warm-ups as a senior. We're just inviting injury to happen.

Instead, think of warm-ups as a fun game! During warm-up, we are gifted the opportunity to get mentally ready and bring conscious awareness to the control of our breath and our body.

Wall Leg Stretch

The wall leg stretch is a fantastic exercise to lengthen and stretch the hamstrings, calves, and lower back.

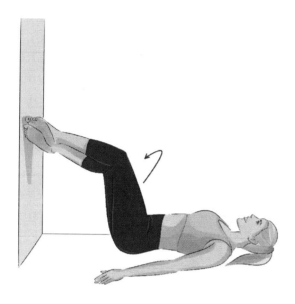 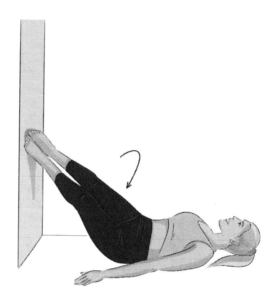

Starting Position

Lie on your back on a comfortable surface or mat, placing your feet comfortably against the wall at a 45-degree angle.

Pose 1

As you inhale, use your toes to guide you and turn to the right with both legs. Exhale freely and maintain the position for five seconds.

Pose 2

Release to the starting position. Now repeat the same movement on the left side with both legs. Maintain for five seconds.

Repeat the left and right movements five times on each side for ten total movements. Only go as

far as you comfortably can. If this feels relaxing to you, continue—sometimes, I continue this until my whole lower body feels loose and relaxed.

Tips:

- If you have back or pelvic pain, be careful not to overextend on this exercise. Turn only left or right at a comfortable range for you.

- Keep your head against the floor when you do this. Make sure your spine is aligned and the weight is fully dropped, like you're melting into the floor.

Wall Staff Pose

This exercise stretches your back and aligns your shoulder and lower back for better posture. It can also be used as a great resting position after a workout.

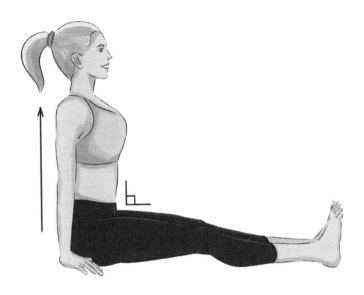

Starting Position

Lean your head and butt firmly against the wall. Place your hands to the side with fingers pointing forward and toes pointing up.

Pose 1

Extend your spine. Imagine you are becoming as tall as possible without forcing it.

Stay here for up to thirty seconds.

Tips:

- Remember to keep your toes pointed up.

- A variation of this is to place your hands on your lap. You may recognize this pose in the Egoscue method. Make sure your shoulders are aligned between the left and right, and maintain your contact with the wall throughout.

Shoulder Arm Stretch

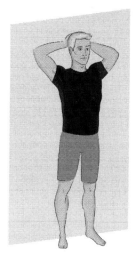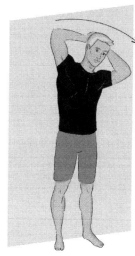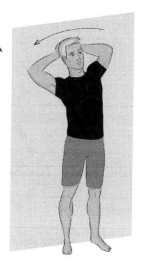

Starting Position

Stand against the wall with your hands at the back of your head.

Pose 1

Use your hands and guide your head to the left. Take a breath here.

Pose 2

Now, guide your head with your hands to the right. Take a breath here.

Perform Poses 1 and 2 for ten reps each for a total of twenty.

Knee Stretch

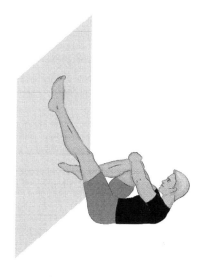

Starting Position

Lean both legs against the wall comfortably.

Pose 1

As you inhale, bend your right leg and hold your knee with both hands. Raise your head as you do this. Take three breaths here.

Pose 2

Now repeat for the other side.

Perform Poses 1 and 2 for six reps.

Hugging Knee Pose

A gentle hip opener and a back stretch that can be both relaxing and rejuvenating.

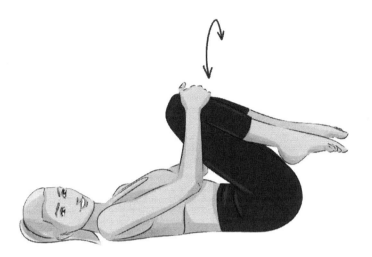

Knees to Chest: Lying on the floor, bend your knees and bring them toward your chest.

Hold Your Knees: Reach up to grab the outer edges of your knees with your hands.

Gentle Rock: If it feels good, you can gently rock from side to side or up and down, massaging your back against the floor.

Hold and Release: Stay in this pose for anywhere from thirty seconds to a few minutes, depending on your comfort. To come out of the pose, gently release your feet and put them down on the mat.

Tips:

Once you're in the pose, take deep breaths and relax. Let the gravity help deepen the hip opening, but don't force anything.

Wall Spine Stretch

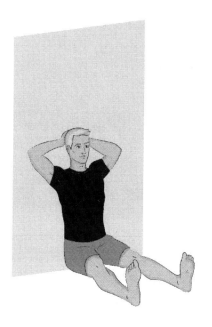 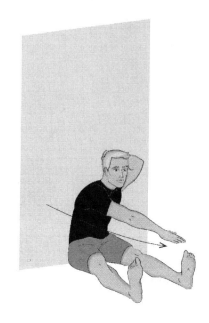 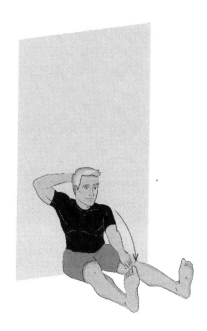

Starting Position

Sit against the wall with your hands gently holding the back of your head.

Pose 1

As you inhale, take your right hand and extend it as far as you comfortably can to the left foot. Exhale freely and maintain the position for five seconds.

Pose 2

Release to the starting position. Now repeat the same movement with your left hand extending to your right foot. Exhale freely and maintain the position for five seconds.

Repeat Poses 1 and 2 for a total of five reps each (ten total). Remember to place your other unextended hand back to the head for an extra upper body stretch.

Child's Pose

A restorative yoga posture that promotes relaxation and stretches the back.

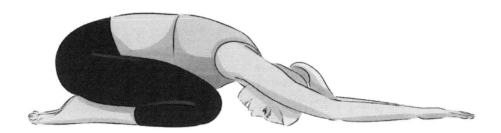

Start on All Fours: Begin in a tabletop position with your wrists under your shoulders and your knees under your hips.

Sit Back: Push your hips back toward your heels, lowering your torso between your thighs.

Extend Arms: Stretch your arms out in front of you, palms facing down on the floor.

Rest Your Forehead: Bring your forehead to the ground.

Relax: Breathe deeply and relax in this position, allowing your back to stretch and your mind to calm.

Hold: Stay in this pose for up to a minute. Sometimes I stay here for a few minutes because it feels so wonderful!

Checking for Trigger Points

One thing you should look into if you're not seeing improvement or feeling good when you do these warm-up exercises... or if you have ongoing pain: check for trigger points (TrPs). If you have active TrPs, exercising the muscle does not solve the problem. In this case, I highly recommend The Trigger Point Therapy Workbook by the late Clair Davies. Using this guide, you will find referral TrPs, which means the source of the TrP is actually far away from the site of pain. Resolving these TrP taut bands usually brings relief.

It bears repeating: If you have muscles ridden with TrPs like I did, you must first get rid of those TrPs. But what comes later is a weak TrPs-free muscle. This is where Pilates comes in. The ability of Pilates to exercise all the slow and fast-twitch muscle fibers and to control smaller muscles that regular exercises don't stimulate to the same level is how I trained my weak muscles to become stronger. With TrPs, our goal is to 1) clear any trigger points in your muscles and then 2) use low-risk, low-impact but efficient exercise movements like Pilates to regain strength. By doing it in this order, you will become tension-free and stronger.

You can check for trigger points by pressing on the points where they exist as in Clair Davies's book. A trigger point will replicate the pain pattern you've been experiencing, and resolving the knot usually resolves the corresponding symptoms. For example, pressing on the lower abdominal wall recreates my pelvic pain, and pressing on my sternocleidomastoid (SCM) muscle can replicate arm pain. In this case, knowing where to find each TrP by reading *The Trigger Point Therapy Workbook* saved my life.

CONTROL AND BALANCE

Joseph Pilates originally chose the name "Contrology" to describe Pilates because he believed his system used the mind to control the body. In this context, "control" means the conscious, deliberate movement and command over one's body.

That's why the exercises in Pilates or Contrology are not about doing rapid, high-repetition sets but rather about performing slower, precise movements with full muscular control.

This gives us a true balance between control, strength, and flexibility.

By controlling our movements with this conscious awareness, we increase your balance awareness, encourage smoother movements, and give an opening to better posture all at the same time.

This section includes exercises that improve your control focus of the movements.

Balance Check

Without stability, bad form can cause injuries and repetitive stress to your whole body. That's why we want to perform all exercises in a stable manner. As you gain stability, everything you do will feel more balanced. We'll call this "balance awareness."

The first step in balance awareness is your feet.

BALANCE CHECK INSTRUCTIONS

1   Stand straight in front of a mirror facing the wall.

2   Feel the alignment of both your feet. Are they properly aligned, or is one foot in front of the other? Are your toes pointed forward with a slight outward tilt? This is the natural alignment of the feet:

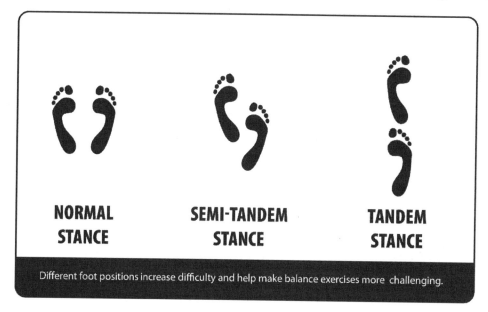

NORMAL STANCE   **SEMI-TANDEM STANCE**   **TANDEM STANCE**

Different foot positions increase difficulty and help make balance exercises more challenging.

3   Now, feel the weight of your body on your feet. Where is the point of center? Is it toward your toes? Or are you always "on your heels?" Or always "tip-toeing" around? The center of weight should be toward the center of your foot, straight down from the ankles.

4   Stop here, take a breath, and feel your weight distribution—it should be balanced fifty-fifty on both feet. Imagine your spine passing down toward your knees and down to your ankles. The image below shows all the alignments you can build awareness around: the head controlled by the neck, the shoulders, the core and hips, your knees, and your feet.

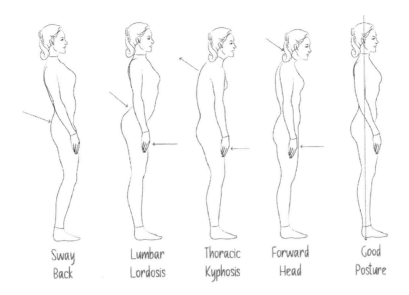

Sway Back | Lumbar Lordosis | Thoracic Kyphosis | Forward Head | Good Posture

5 Use a mirror and look directly at your alignment from head to toe. Turn sideways and look now. How does your body feel? With your face forward, feel the weight distribution on your feet. Take three breaths here and just feel your body. Imagine a smooth line that goes from the top of your head down your spine and through your feet into the ground. Here are some examples of common dysfunctions:

Don't worry about getting it 100 percent right. Just being aware of this will increase your ability to correct any postural issues over time. This exercise trains your mind to become aware of your body's alignment as you go about your day.

The Monkey

This is an Alexander technique designed to build spinal awareness.

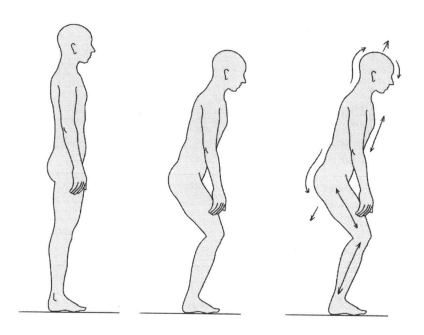

THE MONKEY INSTRUCTIONS

1   You're in a standing position. Come to your full height by allowing your neck to release to let your head go forward and up and your back to lengthen.

2   Now, think of releasing your buttocks muscles outward and downward as you bend your knees.

3   As your butt draws down and its muscles let go, think of releasing the front of your hip joints, behind your knees, and the front of your ankles. I think of this as my head leading the spine to lengthen my lower legs.

4   Allow your knees to release from your lower back, so now you're bending a bit forward but still with a straight spine. This should give you much more freedom and release in your thighs, and you will feel strength in your lower back and pelvic area. Basically, you're lengthening your back while bending your knees. This is great for lower back pain. Hang out here for a few seconds.

5   Using your leg muscles and hip muscles, push yourself back to standing.

6   Try doing three monkeys slowly with full body awareness.

Hip Circles

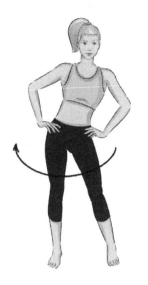 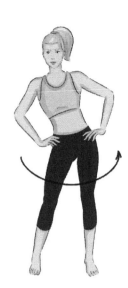

1 Stand with your feet hip-width apart and

   place your hands on your hips.

2 Rotate your hips outward (clockwise), keeping
   the upper body stable. Circle as far as you can
   while maintaining stability. Perform 10 circles.

3 Now rotate your hips inward (anticlockwise),
   keeping the upper body stable. Circle as
   far as you can while maintaining stability.
   Perform 10 circles.

Tips:

Breathe steadily throughout the exercise.

The Wall Roll Up

A beautiful exercise that practices slow and deliberate control of the upper body. Great for your spine.

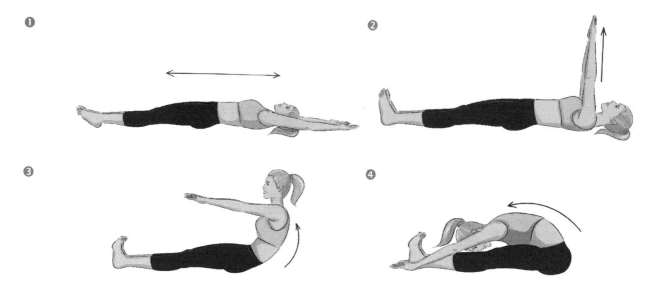

Starting Position

Lie flat and let the weight of your entire body rest on the floor. Stretch your arms straight backward and place your toes against the wall.

The wall is optional in this pose. Use it to help you gain resistance to help with this movement and to keep your legs straight. As you gain flexibility, leave the wall and stretch your hands out further than your toes in the last movement.

Pose 1

As you inhale slowly, bring your arms straight up with your toes pointing upward.

Pose 2

As you exhale slowly, bring your chin down and your head forward.

Pose 3

While exhaling slowly, roll forward as much as you comfortably can and hold for ten seconds. You can do a back-and-forth rock here with

the stretch and see if you can reach just a little further each time.

Repeat the poses four times, and remember to breathe slowly while moving. Use the breath to guide you through the movements. See if you can go further each time.

Tips:

- When lying down (Pose 1), your entire spine must touch the mat or floor and make sure you are fully extended and not tense.

- As you come up, press both legs together and try to keep them against the floor. If you can't, don't sweat the small stuff. Lift them slightly and keep practicing until you can keep both legs against the floor.

- Don't worry if you can't extend all the way down with your head and hands; just stretch as far as you can.

The Spine Stretch

This beautiful pose stretches your entire spine.

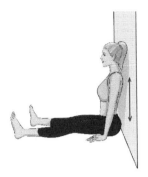 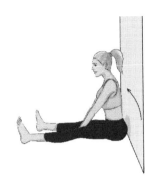 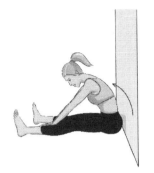 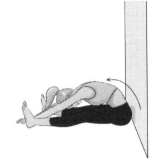

Starting Position

Spread your legs apart as wide as possible while placing your back straight against the wall. Toes pointed upward, rest your palms on each side of the floor.

Pose 1

Begin stretching forward with each "slide" moving forward a little bit until you reach as far as possible.

Pose 2

When you reach your limit, try extending your arms as far as you comfortably can and hold for eight seconds.

Repeat three times and see if you can go a little further each time!

Tips:

- The initial pose uses the wall to remind your body of a straight spine. Starting from a relaxed, straight posture ensures the rest of the exercise goes correctly.

- Keep your head and neck relaxed while extending forward. If you tense the neck and head, it adds more pressure. The whole body, from head to pelvic floor, should feel like a slow, relaxed stretch.

- Take slow, controlled, deep breaths as needed. You can breathe in and out of your mouth for more power to expand and extend your chest area, which will also help your flexibility over time.

- Don't worry if your flexibility is limited when starting out. Go as far as you comfortably can.

Wall Downward Dog

Instead of having hands and feet on the ground, in this modification, the wall adds support against the feet, making the pose more accessible to beginners or those with limitations.

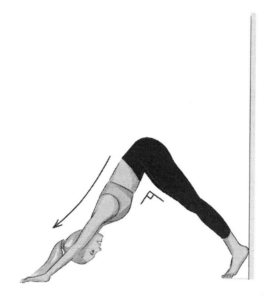

Starting Position

Start with your back against the wall and lean forward, touching the ground with your hands.

Pose 1

Move your hands slowly forward using the wall as support against your feet. Go as far you as you comfortably can.

Pose 2

Now extend your back upward and backward as far as you comfortably can (keeping your head loose) in a straight line down the spine.

Press into the floor with your chest and up into the air with your buttocks. Hold and breathe for fifteen seconds.

> **Tips:**
>
> I inhale as I move forward and exhale as I press onto my feet.

Wall Downard Facing Dog

This variation offers many of the same benefits as the traditional pose but with a different level of intensity and control for the smaller back muscles.

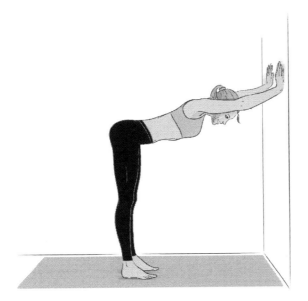 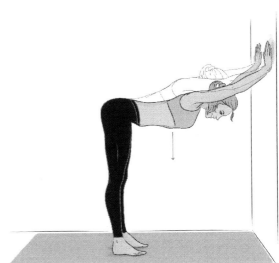

Starting Position

Stand facing a wall, about an arm's length away. Comfortably place your hands on the wall above your head. Slowly slide down with your arms and bow your head to the wall.

Pose 1

Press your chest toward the ground, keeping your ears aligned with your upper arms. Push your hips back, your legs straight, and your heels grounded.

Pose 2

Engage your core and hold for three deep breaths. Return to standing to release.

Repeat three times.

Tips:

- Avoid hyperextension: Be mindful not to lock your elbows or knees. A tiny, soft bend can prevent hyperextension.

- Adjust distance for comfort: Depending on your height and flexibility, you may need to adjust how far you stand from the wall or how high your hands are placed.

- Flexibility considerations: If you're more flexible, you might find that placing your hands lower on the wall (closer to waist height) offers a deeper stretch.

Legs Up the Wall Pose

Using gravity, this pose realigns your hips and feels very relaxing!

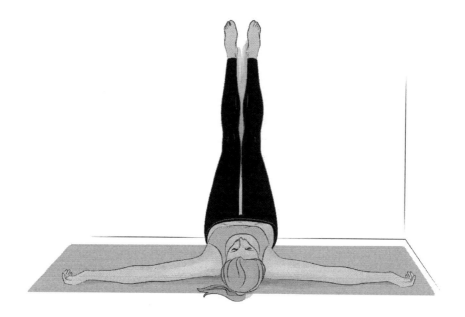

Starting Position

Position your mat perpendicular to the wall to ensure a comfortable base for your back.

Sit sideways against the wall, with one hip touching it.

Pose 1

Swing your legs up onto the wall as you lie back onto the mat. Adjust so your buttocks are close to or touching the wall with your legs straight up.

Pose 2

Place your arms at your sides, palms facing up.

Variations

A variation of this is to put the arms sideways like a cross (pictured) or completely relaxed, extended above your head on the mat.

Relax and breathe deeply, holding the pose for thirty seconds. Sometimes, I stay here for up to a minute.

Release

To exit, bend your knees, roll to one side, and gently push up to a seated position.

Tips:

- You can use a pillow or folded blanket under the lower back or hips for added support if needed.

- This pose with the hands fully extended like a cross is also found in the Egoscue method. It realigns the hips and legs.

Straddle Pose

This movement allows us to stretch both legs wide apart safely using gravity.

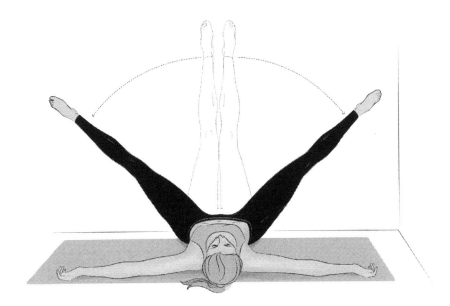

Starting Position

Position your mat perpendicular to the wall.

Sit sideways against the wall with one hip touching it.

Swing your legs up onto the wall as you lie back onto the mat. Adjust so your buttocks are close to or touching the wall.

Pose 1

Extend your legs straight up the wall.

Pose 2

Slowly open your legs into a V shape, letting gravity pull them down toward the floor. Go as far as you can comfortably.

Pose 3

Rest your arms straight down each side. Relax and breathe deeply, holding the pose as long as it is comfortable. I usually hold this for up to a minute because it feels so good.

To exit, gently use your hands to bring your legs back together, then bend your knees and roll to one side.

Tips:

If you can't extend your legs fully straight, don't worry. It's okay to bend them a little and go as comfortably as far as you can with widening.

Standing Side Bend Pose

A simple yet effective exercise giving your sides an amazing stretch.

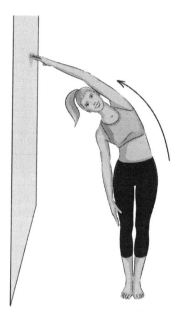

Starting Position

Stand sideways approximately an arm's length from a wall. Plant your feet firmly and closely together.

Pose 1

Extend the arm further from the wall overhead and place that hand on the wall for support. Take a deep breath in, and as you exhale, gently bend your torso for a deep stretch.

Pose 2

At the same time... the opposite arm can be extended alongside and down your body for another stretch. Hold for a few breaths, feeling the stretch along your sides.

Reverse Sides

Turn around and repeat on the opposite side as many times as you like. I do three stretches on each side for about fifteen seconds each.

Tips:

- Ensure you're bending from the waist, not the hips.

- Keep both feet grounded and maintain a soft bend in your knees to avoid locking them.

- Adjust the distance from the wall as needed for comfort.

Garland Pose with Wall

A deep squat that uses the wall for support while giving you a deep stretch of the lower body.

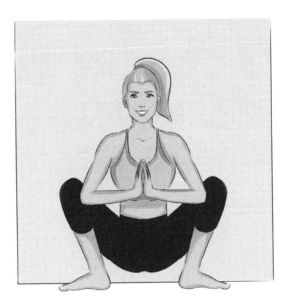

Starting Position

Stand with your back to a wall, feet wider than hip-width apart. Turn your toes out slightly.

Pose 1

Begin to squat down, keeping your heels on the ground if possible. If your heels lift, you can place a folded mat or blanket under them for support.

Allow your thighs to be wider than your torso, pressing your elbows against the inner knees.

Pose 2

Join your palms together in front of your heart. You can press your hips and even lower your back gently against the wall for alignment and support.

Breathe deeply and hold for up to thirty seconds.

To release, press on your feet and return to a standing position.

Tips:

- The wall provides support and helps in maintaining balance.

- Use your arms to push your legs even further out.

- As you get better, you can move away from using the wall. It's a beautiful movement either way.

Standing Backbend Pose

**This is a great way to open the font of the body for release.
Be careful to only go as far as is comfortable.**

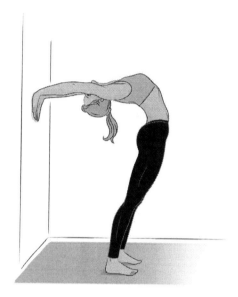

Starting Position

Stand facing away from a wall, about a foot or two away, depending on your flexibility. Your feet should be comfortably apart.

Pose 1

Lean back and place your hands behind you on the wall, fingers pointing down.

Pose 2

Press onto your feet, engaging your thighs and core. Begin to lift your chest upward and arch your back. Allow the head to drop gently backward if comfortable.

Pose 3

Push against the wall with your hands for support and breathe deeply, holding the pose for up to thirty seconds.

To exit, engage your core and slowly lift your torso, returning to a neutral standing position.

Tips:

- You can keep a slight bend in the knees to avoid hyperextension.

- Always move within your comfort range to avoid straining the back and neck.

Wall Butterfly Pose

The force of gravity, combined with the support of the wall, provides a gentle and effective stretch for your adductors and hamstrings.

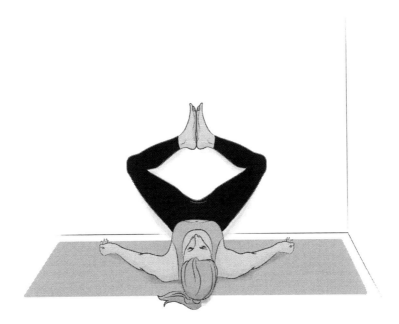

How to Get into a Starting Position (Easy Mode)

Sit on the floor with your buttocks close to a wall, sitting sideways to the wall to your right. As you lean your back to the right, you will automatically raise both legs against the wall.

Pose 1

Allow your legs to gently open, with your heels sliding down the wall toward your pelvis and forming a triangle shape with your legs.

Let both feet come together until they are pressing against each other.

Pose 2

Relax your arms to the floor on each side.

Variation

Bring your hands into a prayer pose.

Relax and breathe deeply, feeling a gentle inner thigh stretch.

To exit, roll to either side and gently extend your legs.

> **Tips:**
>
> Adjust the distance from the wall to change the intensity of the stretch.

Wall Roll Down

This exercise is often used in physical therapy sessions to promote spinal mobility and awareness.

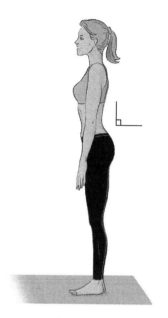 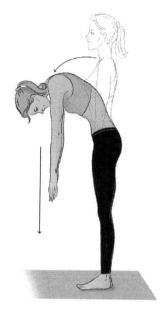 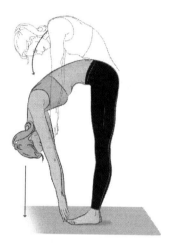

Starting Position

Stand with your back against the wall for posture alignment, both arms comfortably lowered on each side. Your feet should be a few inches away from the wall. Your butt can be touching the wall for another point of reference in your spinal alignment.

Pose 1

Tuck your chin to your chest.

Begin to roll down slowly by lowering your hands to the mat, allowing your back to round as you do so.

If you're having trouble, bend the knees slightly as needed.

Pose 2

Pause for a breath at the bottom with the crown of your head pointing toward the floor.

Slowly roll back up to standing, restacking the spine, and lifting the head last.

Repeat five times.

Tips:

- This exercise promotes spinal flexibility and can be used to relieve tension in the back.

- Bend your knees if needed for comfort and to suit your flexibility.

- As you gain flexibility and can keep your legs and back straight, you no longer need to use the wall. I use it occasionally to check my alignment.

- If your flexibility improves, you can move your hands to hold in your elbows to create even more space to move further down.

CARDIO FOCUS

There are many benefits of cardiovascular exercise. From improved metabolism to improved lung capacity and improved sleep... the list goes on.

If you've heard the term "Pilates body," it's because the following exercises not only use cardio to burn calories, they also strengthen and tone your muscle groups at the same time.

That said...it's important to remember that Pilates is a system developed by Joseph Pilates that involves low-impact exercises designed to strengthen muscles, improve postural alignment, and enhance flexibility. So, while not specifically designed for weight loss, it's a very visible secondary effect.

Best of all, you'll feel stronger, be more flexible, and move with a more aligned posture.

The following exercises burn energy and are designed to be senior-friendly. Of course, if the exercise looks too difficult, consider finding a friend or spotter or even hiring a professional trainer. Don't overdo it.

Wall Leg Raise to Back Kick

This routine activates your glutes and lower back and strengthens your leg muscles.

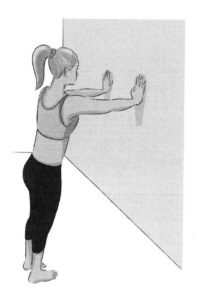 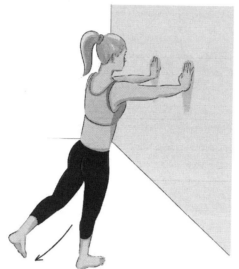 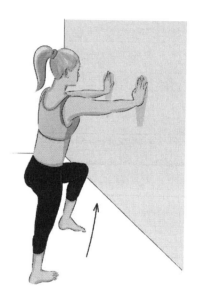

Start Position

Stand upright next to a wall and put both hands on the wall for balance. Stand close enough to easily touch the wall without leaning into it.

Pose 1

Slowly lift your left leg and go as high as you can. Hold this position for two seconds.

Pose 2

With a controlled movement, now move your left leg backward, almost like a slow kick away from the wall. Engage your glute muscles and thighs and go as far as you can. Hold here for two seconds.

Repeat this five times, then switch to the right leg and do a total of ten reps.

Tips:

Use controlled movements rather than relying on momentum.

Wall Plank

The wall plank is more beginner-friendly than a regular blank while still improving your upper body strength and flexibility.

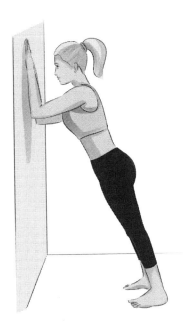

Starting Position

Place your hands and forearms flat against the wall, slightly wider than shoulder-width apart.

Lean In: Walk your feet back and then lean into the wall.

Your body should be at an incline, with your weight supported by your hands and forearms. Ensure your body forms a straight line from your head to your heels.

Hold: Maintain this plank position. Keep your core engaged.

Breathe: Breathe steadily. Avoid holding your breath.

Duration: Aim to hold the plank for twenty to thirty seconds to start, gradually increasing the time as you become stronger.

Return: To come out of the plank, walk your feet toward the wall and stand upright.

Tips:

- Avoid sagging in the lower back or hiking the hips up. Maintain a straight line.

- Keep your head in a neutral position in line with the spine.

Leg Embrace

This routine activates your glutes and lower back and strengthens your leg muscles.

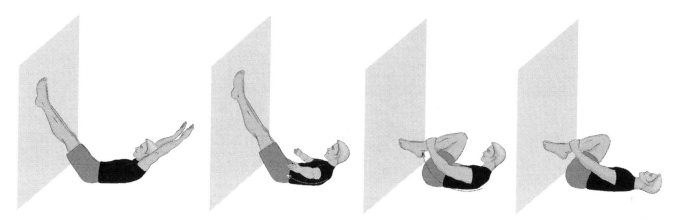

Starting Position

Place both feet against the wall, lying back with your hands extended backward.

Embrace: Weave both hands in a circle toward the wall. Your head should be slightly raised and you should feel like you're extending your body, releasing instead of holding or tightening.

Pose 1

As your hands reach the wall, bend your knees and bring your legs in toward your chest.

Pose 2

Hold your legs near the ankle area. Breathe steadily. Avoid holding your breath.

Duration: Aim to hold here for up to five seconds.

Pose 3

Return to the starting position by releasing the feet. Extend your feet up the wall and your arms back again.

Now, perform this movement for ten reps.

> **Tips:**
> - Being conscious of all the movements here instead of "trying to get it over with" is important to gaining mobility instead of tightening.
> - Keep your head in a neutral position just slightly above the floor.

Wall Calf Raises

This is a great exercise for posture alignment and strengthening the calf muscles.

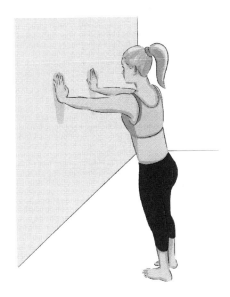 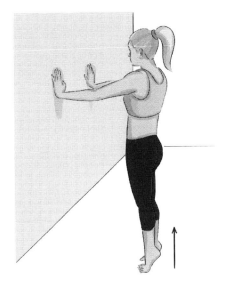

Starting position

Stand facing a wall with feet hip-width apart and arms comfortably extended against the wall.

Pose 1

Place your hands on the wall for balance. As you inhale, rise onto the balls of your feet, lifting your heels as high as possible. Hold for two seconds.

Pose 2

On the exhale, slowly lower your heels back to the ground.

Do ten reps.

Variation

You can isolate each leg and raise only one at a time. Be sure to repeat the same number of lifts for the other calf.

Tips:

The initial pose uses the wall to remind your body of a straight spine.

Wall Twist

A beautiful upper body stretch that loosens the spine, shoulders, and arms.

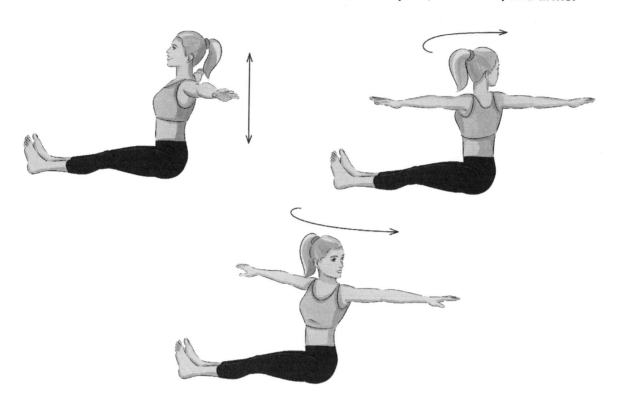

Starting Position

Sit with your legs straight and together on the ground. Feet touching or slightly apart is fine. The wall is optional, but you can put both feet against the wall for balance. Extend your arms out at shoulder height.

Note: The wall is optional if you need help keeping your legs in place and lowered to the floor.

Pose 1

Inhale, turn the body to the right, and extend as far as is comfortable.

Pose 2

Exhale and rotate now to the center, and then turn the body to the left and extend as far as is comfortable.

Repeat eight turns for a thorough stretch of the arms and upper body.

If you're having trouble keeping your legs straight, it's okay to bend them a little bit.

Tips:

- Keep hips stable: Your hips should remain square and facing forward throughout the movement. The twist should come from the thoracic (upper) spine and not the lumbar (lower) spine.

- Stay upright: Ensure you remain tall and avoid leaning forward or backward during the twist.

The Backward Balance

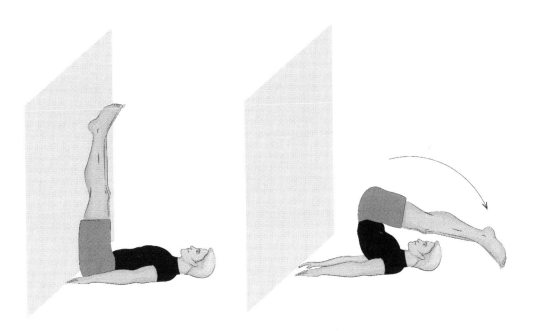

Starting Position

Sit with your legs straight and together on the ground, with the wall to your right. Lean to the right and bring your feet up. Now you've got your legs straight up the wall without any distance from it!

Pose 1

Inhale and bring your legs forward past your head. See if you can touch the floor with your toes while keeping your legs straight. Stay here and take five breaths.

Now, kick your legs back to the wall. Repeat this five times.

Straight-Legged Sit-Ups

A simple and effective core strengthening exercise.

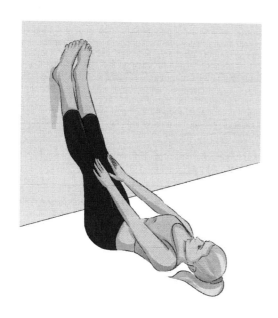 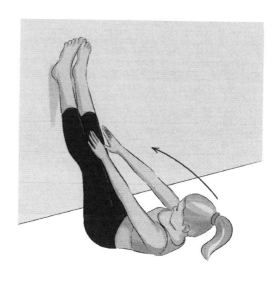

Starting position

Lie on your back with your legs straight up against the wall and your feet together. Place your hands on your knees.

Pose 1

Engage your core and lift your head off the ground, keeping your legs stationary.

Move your hands upward as far as you can comfortably, moving from your core.

Pose 2

Slowly lower back down to the starting position.

Perform ten reps. You can inhale when lowering down and exhale when going upward.

Tips:

When starting out, focus on performing each repetition with good form rather than trying to do as many as possible. Quality reps will be more effective in targeting the right muscles.

Wall Leg Swings

Leg swings are an excellent way to increase hip and leg flexibility and mobility.

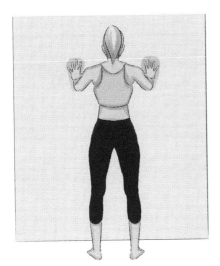 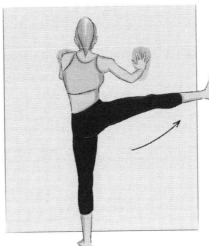 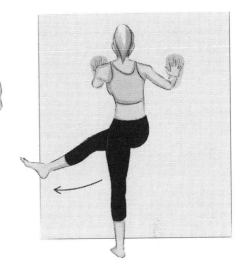

Starting position

Stand straight, facing the wall, and extend your arms to be pushing against the wall. Make sure there is enough space for your legs to swing between you and the wall.

Pose 1

Extend your right leg as far upward to the right as possible while maintaining balance.

Pose 2

Slowly rotate your right leg clockwise, and now swing left. Go as far as you comfortably can.

Repeat Poses 1 and 2 for ten full swings.

Repeat on the left leg for ten swings for a total of twenty reps.

> **Tips:**
>
> • Start with little swings and build up to bigger swings to get accustomed to the exercise.
>
> • You can contract your abdominal muscles to maintain a straight back.

Wall Angels

A popular exercise often prescribed by physical therapists and fitness professionals to address postural issues, particularly for individuals who spend extended periods sitting or working at a desk.

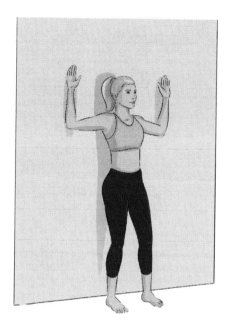 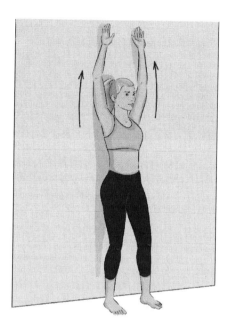

Starting Position

Begin by standing with your entire back pressed against a wall. Your feet should be about hip-width apart and positioned a few inches away from the wall. This stance helps maintain a neutral spine.

Pose 1

Hold your arms up with a 90-degree angle at your elbows. Use the wall to guide you and for resistance support.

Pose 2

Extend your arms upward. Drop back down to Pose 1.

A variation is to extend upward, and then bring your hands together in a prayer pose, pointing to the sky. Then, drop back down to Pose 1.

Perform ten reps.

Tips:

- If you're having trouble or rehabilitating from an injury, prioritize form over range of motion. As your shoulder mobility improves, the movement may become easier.

- As you gain strength and postural awareness, you can do this without wall support.

Wall Sit-Ups

Using the wall, we can add support while improving strength, balance, and coordination of the core muscles.

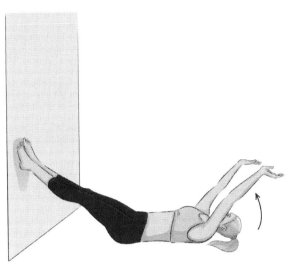 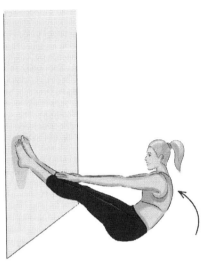

Starting Position

Begin by lying down, feet facing the wall.

Pose 1

Place your feet up against the wall.

Pose 2

Start by raising your arms over your head. Next, engage your core muscles and move your arms toward the wall.

As your hands move above your head, engage your core and raise your head like you are doing a sit-up until you are facing the wall.

Reach your hands as far as you can up toward your feet. You don't have to touch your legs or your feet; just feel the core movement upward and toward the wall.

Return

When finished, return your spine to the floor as you slowly reverse the action by lowering your head and arms to the beginning position (arms still in the air above your head).

Perform ten reps.

Tips:

If you find it difficult to keep your legs straight, you can bend your knees slightly to help with the movement.

Next Steps

"Pilates is not what you get, it is what you give to yourself."[*]
– John Howard Steel

Once you get into the habit of these movements, you won't want to stop. Use the 28-Day Challenge program to stay motivated and on track.

After a while... doing Pilates to feel more flexible, stronger, toned, and more vibrant every day just becomes an addictive habit!

I know that some of you will want to continue on to more advanced exercises, so before we say goodbye, let me direct you to our exclusive pelvic floor Kegels exercise at **wallpilates.org** as taught by Tim Sawyer, a leading physical therapist who worked with Dr. Anderson and Dr. Wise at the Stanford University Medical Center[**]. When you enter your email address to download this free bonus, you'll also be notified of new Pilates books and new workout routines we will release in the future.

You can also scan the following to get your free bonus:

---

[*]   Steel. *Caged Lion: Joseph Pilates & His Legacy*, (p. 181).
[**]   Authors of *A Headache in the Pelvis: A New Understanding and Treatment for Chronic Pelvic Pain Syndromes*.

Additional Resources

Use this URL from the National Pilates Certification Program to find a certified Pilates instructor:

https://nationalpilatescertificationprogram.org/NPCP/NPCP/Directory/CertifiedTeachersList.aspx

Joseph Pilate's original exercise book:

Return to Life through Contrology

The personal life of Pilates from the perspective of one of his students and close friend, John Howard Steel:

Caged Lion: Joseph Pilates & His Legacy

The philosophy and principles of Pilates:

First published in 1934, this book includes Joseph Pilates' early twentieth-century philosophies, principles, and theories about health and fitness:

Your Health: A Corrective System of Exercising that Revolutionizes the Entire Field of Physical Education

Citations

Images used in this book: Free license from Freepik.com.

Disclosures

Some of the links provided in this book are affiliate links, which help you jump to the exact URL of the resource you're looking for at no additional cost to you.

Made in the USA
Columbia, SC
27 November 2024